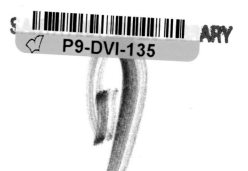

The Complete
Reiki
Tutor

*A structured course to achieve
professional expertise*

Tanmaya Honervogt

This book is dedicated to Lucia,
my beloved mother.

An Hachette UK Company
www.hachette.co.uk

First published in Great Britain in 2008 by Gaia,
a division of Octopus Publishing Group Ltd
Carmelite House, 50 Victoria Embankment
London EC4Y 0DZ
www.octopusbooks.co.uk
www.octopusbooksusa.com

This edition published in 2018

Distributed in the US by Hachette Book Group
1290 Avenue of the Americas
4th and 5th Floors
New York, NY 10104

Distributed in Canada by Canadian Manda Group
664 Annette St., Toronto, Ontario, Canada M6S 2C8

ISBN: 978-1-856-75378-4

A CIP catalogue record for this book is available
from the British Library.

Printed and bound in China

10 9 8 7 6 5 4 3 2 1

All reasonable care has been taken in the preparation of this book, but the information it contains is
not meant to take the place of medical care under
the direct supervision of a doctor. Before making
any changes in your health regime, always consult a
doctor. Any application of the ideas and information contained in this book is at the reader's sole
discretion and risk.

Contents

Introduction

Reiki is a simple and natural healing technique, rediscovered at the end of the 19th century by Dr Mikao Usui, who developed the healing method as it is still used today. When using Reiki you transfer Universal Life Energy for healing. Once you have become a channel for this energy, through taking the three degrees, you feel concentrated life energy flowing through your arms and hands of its own accord. You retain this ability for the rest of your life. Reiki can be learnt by anyone who is open and willing to let this healing energy flow through them.

Learning Reiki

Reiki is easy to learn and simple to use, and you can practise it anywhere, at any time: you always have your hands with you. You can also easily integrate Reiki into your daily activities and use it at home, at work or while travelling. Reiki supports whatever needs healing – whether emotional, physical, mental or spiritual healing. This powerful natural energy is available at all times and sustains our lives every day. Reiki works in a holistic way, helping you to promote better health and well-being. Its energy heals, harmonizes and balances the whole person.

Learning Reiki is particularly useful for people working in medical, psychological and caring professions, such as nurses, doctors, psychotherapists, chiropractors, dentists, masseurs, teachers and carers, whether of the young or the elderly. When you work with people, Reiki enhances the quality of your healing care. It complements the methods of all styles of healing, including orthodox medical treatment, natural therapies, massage and psychotherapy. It can be given in conjunction with any treatment and is not intrusive.

The most profound meaning of Reiki is to develop yourself as much as you can, to grow spiritually and finally become at one with the whole. The inner space from which you transmit Reiki energy in a treatment or attunement always encompasses love, compassion and respect for yourself and for the receiver. Healing always happens from the heart, which creates a loving and accepting space that we share with each other. To live these qualities and just 'be' them is the ultimate significance of Reiki.

Tanmaya's Reiki lineage

Tanmaya Honervogt's lineage goes back directly to the source of Reiki. She trained with one of the few Masters initiated by Hawayo Takata, who introduced Reiki to the West. She is a link in the chain of spiritual tradition started by Dr Usui, the founder of Reiki. Her methods of teaching adhere to the nine elements of the Usui tradition, which include the original Reiki symbols, hand positions and energy attunements.

Tanmaya's lineage can be shown thus:

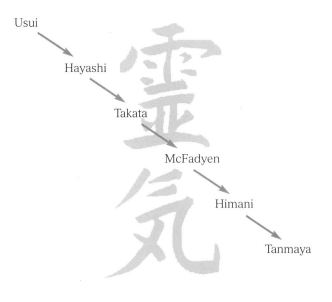

Usui

Hayashi

Takata

McFadyen

Himani

Tanmaya

You can use Reiki in any everyday situation, whether at home or at work, to channel healing energy, which in turn harmonizes the whole body, mind and emotions.

How to use this book

This book is for all those who are interested in healing and spiritual development, regardless of whether you are new to Reiki or already an established Reiki practitioner or teacher.

This book gives you a complete, fresh view of this exceptional healing method, covering all the vital aspects of the healing art of Reiki. It provides you with a thorough foundation, from self-treatment to treating others, and works through the teaching content of all three levels of training (First, Second and Third Degrees). All the necessary hand positions showing how to treat common ailments and possible emotional causes of illness are examined and illustrated. It also explores the spiritual aspects of Reiki in depth, enabling practitioners at all levels to find new inspiration for their personal and spiritual development, and permitting fresh insights that can be applied to personal issues as well as life phases that are common to all of us.

The book looks at the constant interaction between body, psyche and emotions, and explains the connection between negative thought patterns and physical disease, and how we can heal ourselves positively, incorporating Reiki. Our natural state as human beings is to be healthy and contented, and Reiki can heal, harmonize and balance us to that end.

This book gives you the complete teaching of Reiki, to support you and enable you to develop an aware, loving and enjoyable relationship with yourself, with others and

LEARNING STEP BY STEP

The Reiki routines are all broken down into a series of steps, each one accompanied by an illustration showing you exactly where to place your hands on yourself, if you are self-treating, or the person you are treating.

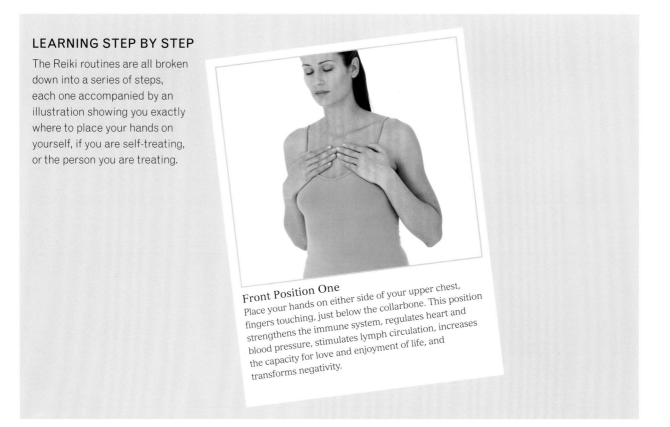

Front Position One
Place your hands on either side of your upper chest, fingers touching, just below the collarbone. This position strengthens the immune system, regulates heart and blood pressure, stimulates lymph circulation, increases the capacity for love and enjoyment of life, and transforms negativity.

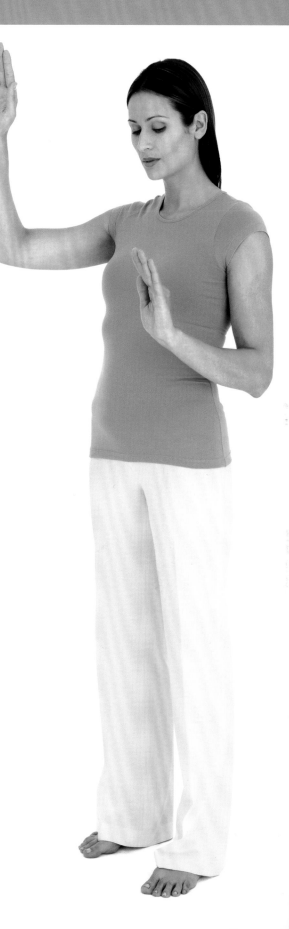

with life itself. It offers guidance for your spiritual journey and contributes to your personal well-being, always remembering that Reiki power is an essential implement to reconnect you with your resources and return you to your true essence. It enables you to finally wake up to your own truth, to be 'who you really are': a divine being (spirit), having a precious human (physical) experience.

Taumaya Honervogt

CAUTION

The treatment positions, exercises and meditations in this book are intended for healing, for relaxation and for enhancing well-being. The author nevertheless wishes to point out that, in the case of illness, a medical doctor or professional health practitioner should always be consulted. The Reiki hand positions described may be applied as a form of treatment additional to any other therapy. Reiki works well with other forms of allopathic medicine, without interfering with the desired end results. It will help counter negative effects and reduce pain in most cases.

Neither the author nor the publishers accept any responsibility for the application of the Reiki method described in this book.

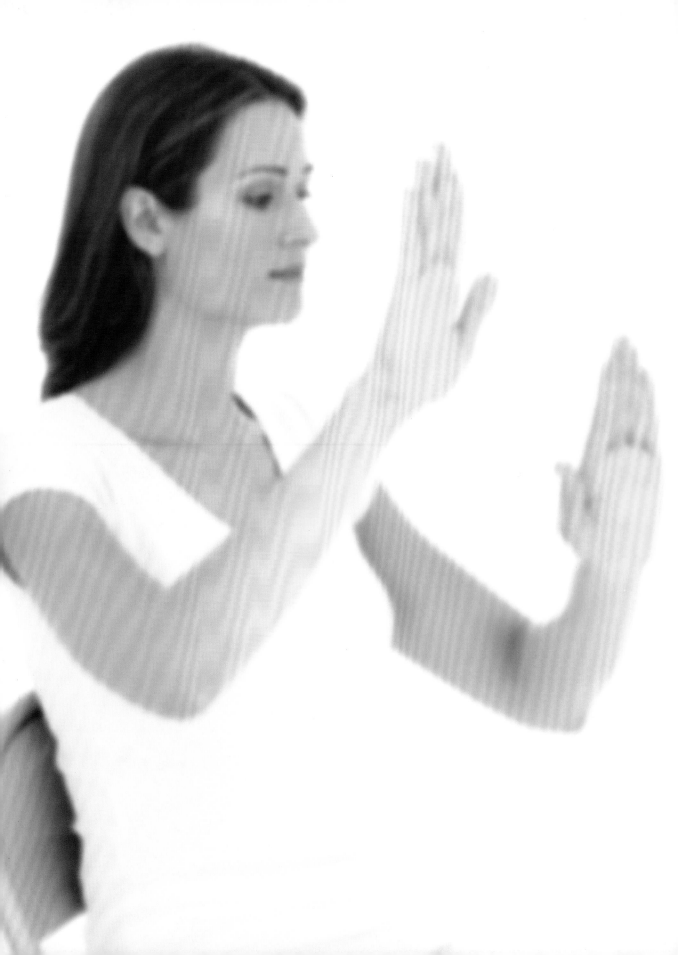

The origins of Reiki

The origins of Reiki go back to ancient Buddhist scriptures, in which a Japanese priest, Dr Mikao Usui, discovered the symbols and mantras, the formula and key, that became the roots and foundations of the Reiki healing system. Following fasting and meditation on a sacred mountain, he found himself in a state of extended consciousness, in which the meaning and use of the symbols and mantras were revealed. Simultaneously, he experienced himself being charged with a healing force. Thus the Usui system of Reiki was born.

The legend of Reiki

The story of how Reiki came into being has been handed down verbally, from Reiki Master to student, in the form of a 'legend'. Reiki was discovered at the end of the 19th century by a Japanese priest, Mikao Usui (1865–1926), who was a Christian minister and president of a small university in Tokyo.

Usui's quest

One day some of his senior students challenged Usui by asking him if he believed in the healing miracles of Jesus, and whether he could demonstrate such a healing and teach it to them. He had no answer, but the incident led to great changes in his life. He dedicated many years to finding out how Jesus and Buddha had been able to heal, on a quest that led him to research both Christian and Buddhist scriptures. He studied Sanskrit – the ancient sacred Indian language – which enabled him to read and understand the original Buddhist writings, and spent considerable time in a Buddhist monastery, where the abbot advised him to meditate in order to find the answers he was seeking.

Enlightenment

Usui embarked on a 21-day meditation and fast on a holy mountain, Mount Kurama, near Kyoto. On the last day he entered an awakening state of consciousness, achieving enlightenment, in which he saw the symbols he had earlier noticed in the Buddhist scriptures. At the same time he received an empowerment and was charged with a powerful healing force. Simultaneously, the application, knowledge and meaning of the symbols and mantras became clear to him. The story goes that he saw a shining light in the sky moving rapidly towards him; it struck him in the middle of his forehead (the third eye) and he found himself in a state of extended consciousness. A great white light then appeared to him, in which he recognized familiar symbols from the Sanskrit sutras (Buddhist scriptures), glowing in gold.

Healing

During his descent from the mountain Usui injured his foot, causing a toe to throb and bleed. When he held his hands around his foot, the bleeding immediately stopped and the pain dissipated. This was his first experience of spontaneous, rapid healing. Later on he healed a young girl's toothache and the abbot's arthritis. He now knew he had finally achieved what he had been seeking: to become enlightened and acquire access to healing energy. He called this energy 'Reiki'.

In 1922 Usui opened his first Reiki clinic in Tokyo. Many people came for treatment and he started to give workshops to share his knowledge. In 1923 there was a devastating earthquake, in which thousands of people were killed, injured or became sick afterwards. Usui gave Reiki to many, and the Meiji emperor honoured him for his work. People showed great respect for his wisdom, knowledge and compassion; he became known as 'Sensei' (teacher), renowned throughout Japan for his remarkable healing skills.

Chujiro Hayashi

A few years before his death, Usui passed his knowledge and teachings on to Dr Chujiro Hayashi (1879–1940), a retired naval officer. Dr Hayashi founded a Reiki clinic in Tokyo that was open to everyone who wanted to receive treatment or learn Reiki. The healers worked in groups, often around the clock, and made home visits. Hayashi left records demonstrating that Reiki reaches the source of the physical symptoms, fills the body with the required energy and restores it to wholeness.

Hawayo Takata

A young Japanese woman, Hawayo Takata (1900–1980), who was suffering from a number of serious disorders, including a tumour, followed an inner call not to have an operation, but to seek healing in Japan. While visiting relatives there she heard about Hayashi's Reiki clinic and went there for several months of treatment, as a result of which she was cured. She was so impressed that she begged Hayashi to teach her Reiki, and he agreed. Takata became his student and stayed with him for a year, after which she returned to her home in Hawaii, where she opened the first Reiki clinic in the West and worked

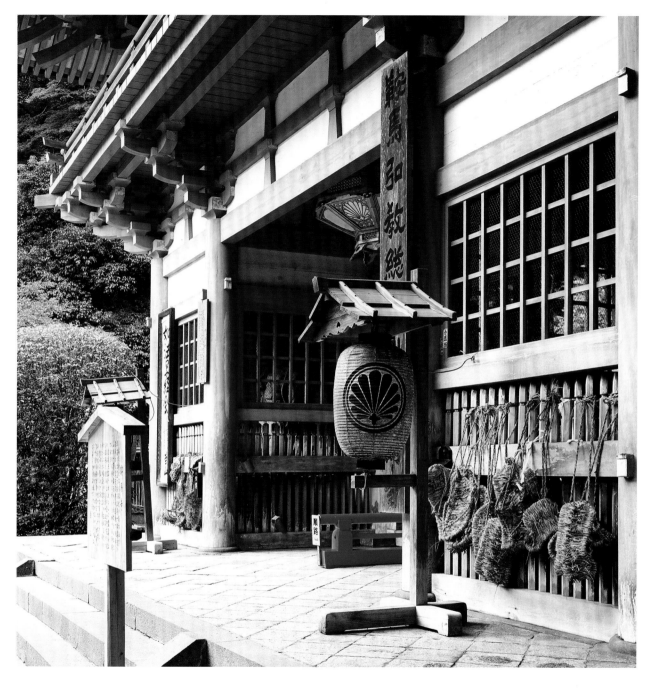

This Buddhist temple, originally founded in the 8th century, is on Mount Kurama. This is the mountain where Usui gained his Reiki healing energy.

successfully as a healer. In 1938 Hayashi visited Takata there and passed on to her the final teachings (the Master level), so that she could teach others.

Mrs Takata also travelled extensively throughout the USA and Canada, treating people and teaching them how to use Reiki for themselves and to heal others. She taught the Reiki system in three levels, or degrees, as she had been taught by Hayashi. In her last years she began to teach the Master level, usually as a form of apprenticeship, in which students worked alongside her for about a year. By her death, she had trained 22 Reiki Masters. Through them Reiki spread widely and became known throughout the Western world.

Dr Usui's story

Mikao Usui was born on 15 August 1865 in the village of Yago in southern Japan. He was a talented and hard-working student, had a wife and two children, and went on to hold several different jobs: government officer, journalist, businessman and secretary to the Mayor of Tokyo.

His life

In the course of his life Usui travelled to the West (the USA and Europe) and also to China to study. He was an honest and dedicated man, interested in history, world religions such as Christianity and Buddhism, medicine and psychology. He was also a seeker and was profoundly interested in meditation (a still state of not thinking, not wanting, not doing – the ultimate state of relaxation) and finding the truth. During his studies he came across ancient Buddhist scriptures, and to be able to read them he learnt Sanskrit. In one of these ancient writings he came across the symbols and mantras that are the key to the Reiki system. After his mystical awakening (enlightenment) on Mount Kurama in 1922, he went on to spend several years devising, practising and teaching the Reiki system.

Recognition

Usui was highly praised by the Meiji emperor of the Meiji Restoration period (1868–1912). During his reign, Japan opened its borders for the first time for many centuries and a new period of openness commenced.

The emphasis of Usui's teaching was not just on physical healing, but also on spiritual awakening. He stressed the importance of living a sincere and spiritual life and adopted 'Principles for Life' from the Meiji emperor, using them as a foundation for his healing work and as guidelines for life, in adherence with the 'Reiki Principles' (see page 21). While he was travelling through Japan, teaching and lecturing about Reiki, he had a stroke and died in 1926 when he was 61 years of age. He is buried with his wife and son at the Shoji Buddhist temple in the suburbs of Tokyo.

Later discoveries

There are numerous stories about Mikao Usui and the history of Reiki. A slightly different picture of Reiki's discovery and development came in the late 1990s from Japan, from two Reiki Masters, the German Master Arjava Petter and his Japanese wife Chetna Kobayashi. Their researches revealed that Usui had been a Buddhist, rather than a Christian, priest. It also became clear that Usui had passed his complete teachings on to 17 people, and not just to Chujiro Hayashi, as stated by Hawayo Takata. It became known that the teaching of Reiki had continued during and after the Second World War and that not all Reiki Masters had been killed in the war.

USUI REIKI RYOHO GAKKAI

In 1926 Mikao Usui founded the Usui Reiki Ryoho Gakkai (Usui Reiki Healing Method Learning Society). This organization was formed to keep Reiki teaching alive, and members of the Gakkai Society have continued to practise and teach Reiki. The first few leaders were taught by Usui and are referred to as 'presidents' of the society. Their names are:

1 Usui
2 Ushida
3 Taketomi
4 Watanabe
5 Wanami
6 Mrs Koyama
7 Kondo

The Gakkai Society is still very active today and holds regular meetings in Tokyo and other locations in Japan. The society's members come together to do meditations for cleansing, purification and strengthening their healing abilities.

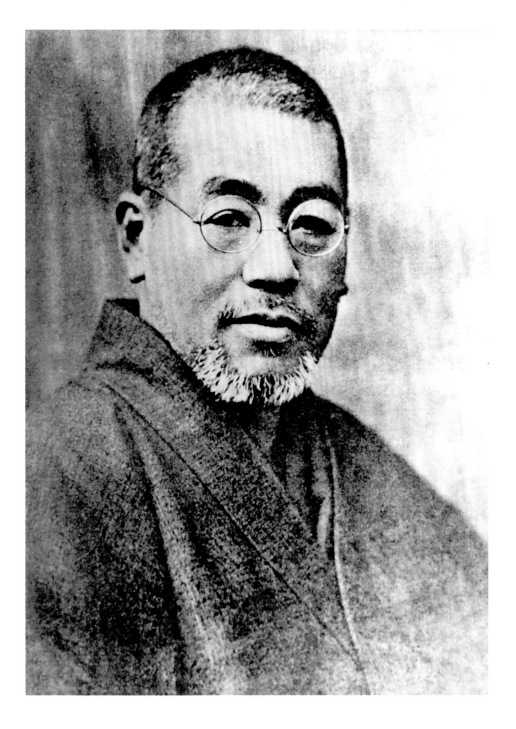

'If Reiki can be spread throughout the world it will touch the human heart and the morals of society. It will be helpful for many people, not only healing disease, but the Earth as a whole.'

Inscription on Dr Usui's headstone

Development of Reiki in the West

Up until Mrs Hawayo Takata's death in 1980, Reiki was known in Japan, the USA, Hawaii and Canada, but her passing led to widespread changes in the small Reiki community. Today, Reiki is known in every country in the world, and there are several thousand Reiki Masters. It is particularly widespread in Spain, Germany, Switzerland, England, Sweden, France, Italy, the USA, Canada, New Zealand, and Australia, and the continents of Asia and Africa are discovering Reiki.

Successors

It is said that Mrs Takata did not leave clear guidance about who her successor was to be. However, her granddaughter, Phyllis Lei Furumoto was recognized by the majority of the 22 Reiki Masters as Takata's successor and founded an organization called the Reiki Alliance in 1983. This association of Masters recognized Phyllis as the Grand Master, and their purpose is to keep the essence of Reiki intact and to support all teachers of the Usui system of Reiki.

Mrs Takata taught Reiki as an oral tradition and usually did not allow her students to take notes. This led to variations in the way Reiki was taught, and so the Masters of the Reiki Alliance decided to standardize the system. They agreed on how the Reiki method should be taught and on exactly what form each Reiki symbol should take. They also accepted the pricing structure that Mrs Takata had set up, as an outward acknowledgement of the value of the priceless gift of Reiki. Living in the West, she realized that her students associated money with value and importance.

Following the tradition of Reiki, only the Grand Master was entitled to pass on the knowledge of Reiki by training other Masters. However, in 1988 Phyllis announced at a meeting of the Reiki Alliance that any experienced Master, who felt ready to do so and take on the complete responsibility for this action, could henceforth teach other Masters. This significant decision opened up the practice of Reiki to many changes concerning the form of its teaching and symbols, and to a worldwide expansion of the healing method.

Hawayo Takata also told many of her Masters to initiate at least one master in their lifetime to ensure that the tradition of the system would continue.

Reiki departures

By the early 1990s an increasing number of Masters had departed from the traditional system taught by Hawayo Takata and agreed by Masters of the Reiki Alliance to work independently. These Masters often changed the way in which Reiki was taught. Some used additional hand positions or added extra symbols and shortened the time of practice between the Reiki degrees. In addition, the way in which the Master degree was taught changed considerably. Some Masters permitted their students to progress through the three degrees very rapidly – sometimes passing all three in a year, a few months or even just a few weeks. With an increased number of new Masters teaching the Reiki First and Second Degrees, Reiki spread rapidly all over the world.

OTHER REIKI METHODS

Rainbow Reiki, Osho Neo-Reiki, Angelic Ray-Key, Blue Star Reiki, Tera-Mai Reiki, Golden Age Reiki, Satya Reiki, Tara Reiki, Vajra Reiki, Braha Satya Reiki, Dorje Reiki, Imara Reiki, Johrei Reiki, New Life Reiki, Reido Reiki, Reiki Plus, Reiki Tummo, Saku Reiki, Ascension Reiki, Amanohuna Reiki, Buddho-Enersense, Ichi Sekai Reiki, Mahatma Reiki, Jinlap Maitri Reiki, Lightarian Reiki, Mari-el, Medicine Dharma Rei Kei, Reiki-Ho, Raku Kei Reiki, Usui-Do Reiki and Sun Li Chung Reiki.

Reiki systems

For the past 20 years new developments and Reiki systems have appeared in the West, although they are all based on the original Usui system. Their founders often incorporated new symbols and different attunements, as well as new teaching styles and their own personal flavours, sometimes adding other features, such as angels, crystals, ascended masters, Buddhist meditation or shamanism.

Different systems

These healing systems, while legitimate, are not the Reiki that Mrs Takata brought from Japan to the West. The changes created a different energy from the original Usui Reiki. They use the word 'Reiki' for identification, and perhaps to benefit from the reputation of the original Usui system. Here is a selection of the existing ones:

Reiki Jin-Kei Do

The Japanese word *Jin* means compassion, while *Kei* means wisdom and *Do* signifies path or way. This form of Reiki emphasizes the spiritual, using the system as a path for enlightenment, as well as for healing. Its Eastern lineage originates from Usui, Hayashi, Tekeuchi (a student of Hayashi) and Dr Ranga Premaratna, its current head. The teaching methods contain many Buddhist practices and meditations because its Masters are often Buddhists.

Seichem Reiki

The lineage of this method goes back to Dr Barbara Weber Ray, and was founded by Patrick Ziegler, one of her students. It is taught over five main degrees and uses a combination of Usui Reiki and other forms from Egypt, with some additional symbols.

Karuna Reiki

Formed by William Lee Rand in the USA in 1993, this system is based on new healing symbols, which are channelled. Its attunement process is different from Usui Reiki, using one Usui symbol, two Tibetan symbols and nine new symbols. It can be taught at a practitioner level for students who want to use it in their healing practice, but is mainly taught at the Reiki Master and teacher level.

Usui Tibetan Reiki

This system is a combination of traditional Usui Reiki, Raku Kei Reiki and its founder William Lee Rand's own teaching. It is taught at four degrees with a different attunement system from traditional Usui Reiki, although it also teaches the traditional Usui Reiki system to Masters.

Usui Shiki Ryoho Reiki

This is the traditional Usui system of Reiki healing, from the lineage of Usui, Hayashi, Takata up to Phyllis Lei Furumoto and any other of the 22 Reiki Masters initiated by Hawayo Takata. Phyllis and Paul Mitchell set up 'The Office of Grand Master', which has outlined important aspects of the teaching, such as healing practice, personal growth, spiritual discipline and the nine elements (oral tradition, spiritual discipline, history, principles, class structure, money, initiation, symbols and treatment) of the Usui system of Reiki. It is taught in three degrees and teaches four symbols. The traditional Usui Reiki is used by Masters who belong to the Reiki Alliance, and by some independent Reiki Masters.

Other branches of Reiki

There are many other forms of Reiki, and all have their own value. To find the right system for you, trust your intuition and choose the one that attracts you the most.

Reiki lineage

To keep the pure energy of Reiki intact, it is important that the lineage of the Master you train with can be traced to the source of Reiki – whether to Usui, Hayashi or Takata. In this way there is a connection between all the Masters. To give an example, the author, Tanmaya Honervogt, is an independent Reiki Master-Teacher, teaching the traditional Usui system of Reiki healing, and receives her lineage directly from Usui, via Hayashi, Takata and Mary McFadyen (see page 6).

Diluted energy

If a lineage is diluted by Masters from other healing systems, the receiver is not acquiring the 'real thing': the pure energy of the Reiki system. For instance, the attunement might merely be a ritual and might lack the spiritual depth it should have. A Master-Teacher with a diluted lineage can transmit energy and teach a healing system, but it will not be the same as the pure energy of Reiki. A Reiki student trained in the First Degree by a Master from the Usui system (Usui-Hayashi-Takata lineage), and then later in the Second Degree by another Master whose lineage is diluted, connects with a different energy, and this will impact on his or her healing; the quality of the Reiki received in the First Degree (with the real Reiki) will also be polluted. The Reiki energy that flows after taking First and Second Degree classes can only be 'pure' if the lineage of all the Masters involved has been uninterrupted by other healing systems.

Reiki today and its importance

Reiki is a dynamic energy. This energy has different names, depending on cultural background (see page 26), but the most commonly known is probably the Japanese word *Ki*. Since Einstein and the discovery of quantum physics, it has been known that everything that exists is energy: 'Energy is all there is.' The only difference is that physical matter (such as a table, chair or car) and unseen energy (sound, light, radio waves or radiation) vibrate at different frequencies and rates. Science has now proved that an invisible energy flows through and connects all living things.

In 1961 the Russian scientist Semyon Kirlian developed a machine to make this 'unseen energy' visible by taking a photograph of it. Tests were carried out on people before and after they had received a Reiki treatment, and it was found that the frequency of the energy was higher when healing energies had been applied. Kirlian photographs also demonstrated that this energy was formed in harmonious patterns.

The need for healing

We are living in a time where healing is needed more than ever. The planet needs it, as do all living beings. Healing is a form of love and comes from the heart, through which we are all interconnected. Reiki opens a space where we can leave our separateness behind; we can connect with what we really are – true essences – and make that inner space available to feel Oneness.

Kirlian photographs have revealed that the nature of the 'unseen energy' that all living things possess can be positively influenced by the application of Reiki treatments.

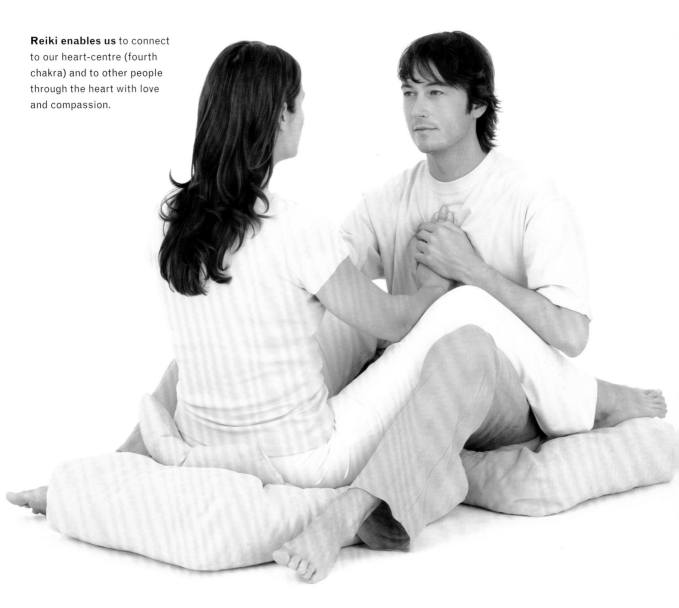

Reiki enables us to connect to our heart-centre (fourth chakra) and to other people through the heart with love and compassion.

Reiki is important today because we can use it to heal and love ourselves. We need to take responsibility for our own lives and what we attract into them. We need to think of ourselves as being lovable, and be grateful for what we already have. By treating ourselves with Reiki, we can start valuing ourselves. By giving Reiki to others, we remember that we are not separate individuals and that we can share the love we have.

The Reiki community

Today Reiki is known in every country in the world, and there are several thousand Reiki Masters. Some have formed organizations, while others work independently. The Reiki Alliance now has almost 1,000 member Master-Teachers. Most countries are members of national Reiki organizations (see page 251) and hold regular meetings and yearly gatherings for Masters and Reiki practitioners.

Reiki Outreach International (ROI) was founded by Mary McFadyen in 1990 and has more than 2,000 members worldwide. Its aim is to address world issues, such as war, natural catastrophes and epidemics, to help, heal and change those situations for the best possible outcomes. Practitioners, either alone or in a group, focus on chosen themes and send healing energy to situations of difficulty anywhere on the planet. Many Reiki students like meeting in small groups, called 'Reiki sharings'. These are organized locally, either on a regular basis (say, once or twice a month) or as and when needed.

The Reiki precepts and principles

These principles were adopted by Usui from the Meiji emperor of Japan. Usui became aware that if someone really wants to change their life, they need to take responsibility for what they create in their life and participate in their own healing process. He passed on these principles as 'guidelines for life'.

Understanding and using the principles today

Part of the spiritual discipline of Reiki is to work with the principles daily. On Usui's headstone it is stated that the student should understand these guidelines in depth, for life, and every day, morning and evening they should

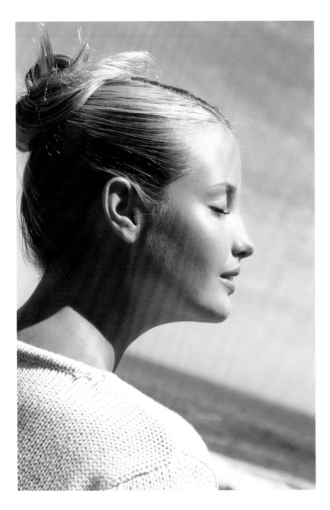

contemplate and chant them. Although these principles are more than 80 years old, they still carry an important message for all. They go deeper than their literal meanings, and meditating on each one helps the student explore their significance.

'Just for today'

This is an instruction to live in the present moment – the only time there is. Past and future do not exist. The mind is forever wandering, keeping itself occupied with thoughts of past or future imaginings. Instead, we need to become aware of the present. There are helpful meditations to achieve this; for example, the Buddhist meditation to watch your ingoing and outgoing breath. You can also ask yourself questions to bring your attention back to the present, such as: 'What is happening right now inside me?', 'What am I thinking?', 'Is my body relaxed?', 'What do I feel?'

'Just for today do not anger'

Anger is a powerful energy and we must not use it destructively. It is often a reaction when our expectations are not met or we feel hurt. Anger can be triggered by a minor incident and the real reason may be unconscious. Those who stimulate our anger may not necessarily be its main cause. Beneath each angry feeling lies a deeper layer of being hurt. Do not feel guilty about anger. First, acknowledge it and take charge of it. Second, recognize the cause. Third, address it and deal with it appropriately, without causing harm. We need to give ourselves permission to release angry feelings. Using Reiki and meditation techniques will help you gain understanding and practise forgiveness.

Meditation can help bring you to an awareness of the here and now – an essential Reiki precept – as well as enabling you to confront and dissipate the destructive power of anger.

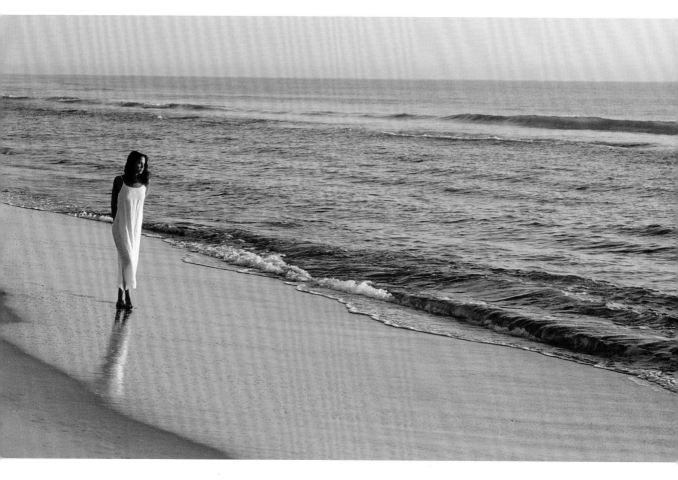

'Just for today do not worry'

What do we usually worry about? Things that may go wrong in the future and things that went wrong in the past. Our worry is linked with fear of the unknown. Worry is a thought pattern, a habit, which results from feeling separate from others and from the universe. It is a negative belief that prevents us from trusting ourselves. Worrying does not lead anywhere. As soon as we realize that being anxious never helps, we can drop it. Whatever problem you are facing, do the best you can and then let go and trust.

Reiki can calm your anxious mind and relax your body; in that way it strengthens your trust in yourself. This lets you surrender to events, knowing that in the end everything will work out for the best. Even if things are unpleasant, later you might realize that actually an important experience took place and the unwelcome event was a 'blessing in disguise'. Through Reiki, meditation practice and prayer we learn to trust the process of life, and become aware that life knows better than us and always cares about us. We are loved by 'God' and by life itself.

Worry is another form of negative energy that Reiki seeks to address. Through the mental calm and physical relaxation that Reiki brings, you will learn to put your trust in the process of life.

THE REIKI PRINCIPLES

The most common form from the Reiki Alliance:

- Just for today do not anger.

- Just for today do not worry.

- Honour your parents, teachers and elders.

- Earn your living honestly.

- Give thanks to every living thing.

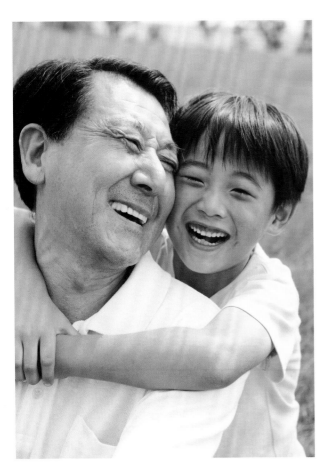

Showing your parents respect and appreciation for all they have done for you, and communicating your love and caring for them, provides a strong basis for healing and happiness.

'Honour your parents, teachers and elders'

We are all teachers and students of one another. This means paying respect to all those who play a part in our life. We share experiences with and learn from each other, and love and support each other. This principle is about letting every situation teach us something. Respect everyone you meet, and value yourself for the precious gift that you are. We learn so much from our parents and teachers. Even if we do not always agree with their actions, we need to be aware that they were influenced by their own parents. Instead of blaming them, give them understanding and compassion. Show gratitude for the good they have done you, and that you care about, love and respect them. Using Reiki and meditation, we can heal past wounds and misunderstandings, and express our love to those who are important in our lives now.

'Earn your living honestly'

This principle means being honest with yourself, and carrying out your work as well as you can. This includes doing what you want to do and enjoying it. It is important to honour your work and acknowledge yourself by doing your best. This gives you satisfaction, and you will love and respect yourself. If you do a job that you do not like, in the long term you will harm yourself, perhaps even falling ill. To be honest to yourself and others takes courage. This means standing up for yourself, and stopping people from using you or breaking your boundaries. Honesty brings clarity and can be challenging in relationships, as it activates deep encounters with loved ones. We need to own our projections and unfulfilled desires by looking closely at our lives and acknowledging with honesty where we are standing. This way the relationship helps you to grow by valuing and respecting each other. Using Reiki and meditation can support you in gaining clarity about 'what you really want in life' and can help you make changes to move forward in life and in your spiritual development.

'Give thanks to every living thing'

The key to happiness is gratefulness. We can be thankful every moment for what life provides. It is human nature to fall into the habit of taking things for granted. We keep on living through our habits, blind to the wonders of life. But life is always unknown and this makes it an exciting adventure. When we allow ourselves to feel this, we become vibrant with energy and joy. We need to be open to receive the gifts that life offers and trust that it will care for us. Each morning we can be thankful for the new day. Through gratefulness we are in communion with existence, we participate and feel: 'I am alive; I am ready for whatever life offers today, for each new event, even if it seems difficult. I trust that existence loves and supports me in my growth. Life trusts me and I trust life, and life always knows better than me.' With gratitude we develop a humbleness in the sense of 'Thy will be done'. We are willing to surrender; then life itself becomes a prayer. Using Reiki and meditation will help us develop gratitude and a sensitivity to become more conscious when old, ingrained patterns of 'taking things for granted' grip us. We deserve to love, and be loved and showered by, the abundance of existence.

Through Reiki you can awaken a sense of wonder at the world around you and learn to appreciate all the simple pleasures that life has to offer every day.

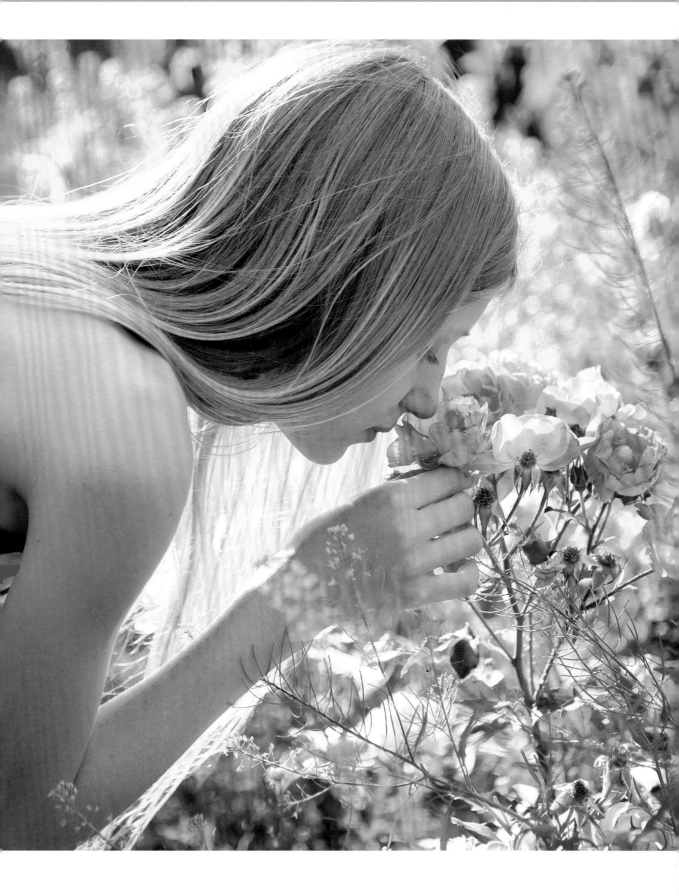

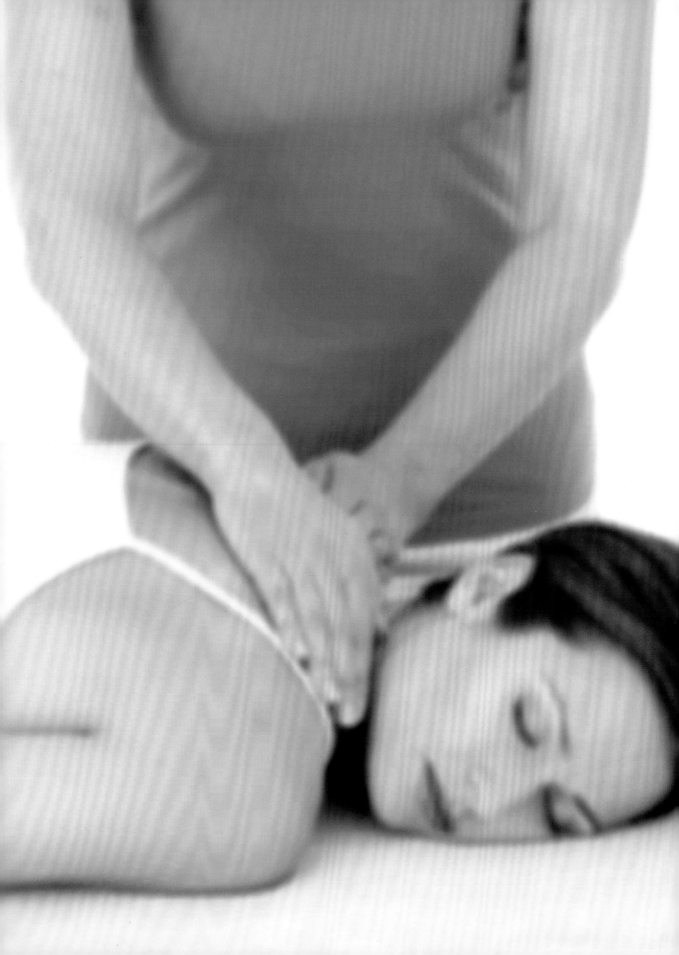

The theory of Reiki

Reiki comes directly from the source of all life and 'aliveness'. According to individual beliefs and the interpretation of language, it comes from the Source, the Vital Force, the Universe or from God. This power manifests itself through Reiki by using an empty vessel (the 'giver') to direct love, light and healing energy to the 'receiver'. Reiki acts like unconditional love, changing and healing whatever it touches; it is the unconditional love of the Universe, of God, automatically acting with love.

What is Reiki?

Reiki is a simple and natural healing method. It is both gentle and powerful, and brings wholeness to the giver as well as to the receiver. Reiki is an ancient hands-on technique, and has no formal connection with any religion, cult, dogma or human belief system.

Definition

The word *Rei-ki* is Japanese, meaning 'Universal Life Energy'. It is defined as being that power which acts and lives in all created matter. The word is in two parts: *Rei* describes the boundless, universal aspect of this energy, while *ki* is the vital life-force energy itself, which flows through all living beings. This energy is described using different words in different cultures. For example, Christians call this vital life force 'Light'; the Chinese know it as *Chi*; the Japanese as *Ki*; the Hindus as *Prana*; and there are many other words, such as *Mana*, bioplasma, 'cosmic energy' and 'life force'. We are all born with this energy; it connects us to all living things and keeps us alive. The closer we can get to its basic form, the more effective it is and the easier it is to use.

How does Reiki work?

Dr Usui developed a method of transferring this Universal Life Energy so that it can be used for healing ourselves and others. 'The attunement process' (see page 52) is the special key to the Reiki system, making it a unique form of healing, different from all other hands-on techniques. To become a 'channel' for Reiki energy, Reiki healers receive an attunement to the Reiki power. This is also called an 'energy-transmission' or 'initiation', and can only be given by a qualified Reiki Master-Teacher. The attunement process usually takes the form of a simple ceremony in which the Reiki Master uses the confidential Reiki symbols and mantras to transmit energy to the student. Each energy-transmission opens up the 'inner healing channel' and attunes the student to its vibrational frequency. This transmission amplifies the flow of energy and heightens the vibratory rate of the body's energy. The energy enters the student's body through the top of the head and flows through the upper energy centres, known as 'chakras'. The energy continues down the arms and leaves the body by radiating out from the hands. Once a student has become a channel for this energy, he or she feels concentrated life energy flowing through the arms and hands of its own accord. The student retains this ability for the rest of his or her life.

Who can learn Reiki?

Reiki can be learnt by anyone who is open and willing to let this healing energy flow through them. Anyone can become a channel for this form of healing, including children. Reiki can be used to complement the healing properties of all kinds of medical practice, both orthodox and alternative, and can be given in conjunction with any other treatment. Because Reiki is a vibrational healing energy, it is not intrusive and will pass through clothing, bandages, braces, plasters, casts and even metal.

What is Reiki healing?

The root of the word 'healing' comes from the word 'whole'. When we are connected to the 'whole', our energy is flowing and we feel alive, vibrant and healthy. As soon as we allow our energy to be drained or blocked by physical, mental or emotional issues, we become ill. Anyone who gives Reiki is being used as a 'channel' for Reiki energy, first to flow through him or her, and second to pass it on to the receiver – the person who needs healing. While touching the body of the sick receiver, the giver becomes a link to the source of healing. Reiki helps us to become reconnected to the source and to the 'whole', to 'God' or the life force. This gentle, powerful 'hands-on' technique brings wholeness to both receiver and giver. You cannot 'overdo' Reiki or give too much of it, because it adjusts itself to the needs of the receiver and restores natural balance in the body.

Through the attunement process, the Reiki student becomes a channel for a vibrational healing energy, which flows through the arms and hands.

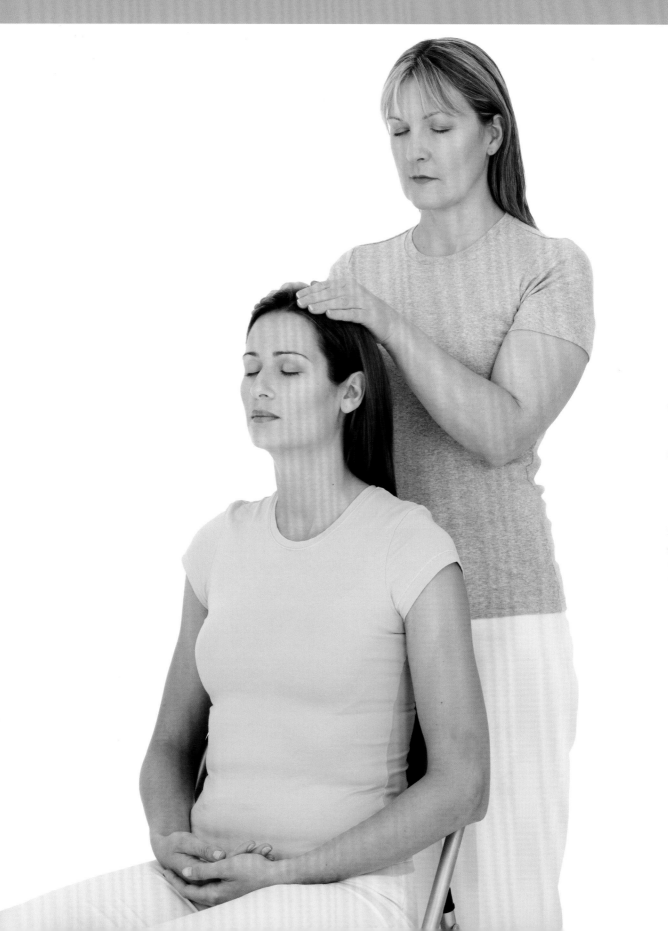

The four levels of Reiki

Reiki affects each person differently, but it always acts wherever the receiver needs it most. It works on the levels of mind, body, emotions and spirit, and produces a deep cleansing effect. It provides deep relaxation, evoking a sense of peace and well-being. Reiki energy is pleasant and holistic, revitalizing body and soul.

On the physical level

Reiki helps a person to sustain physical health by strengthening the immune system. It loosens blocked energy and helps cleanse the body of toxins. It can relieve pain and stress symptoms, and is rejuvenating. Reiki can also replace energy used up in everyday life. If there is too much (or too little) energy in a certain area, that part of the body is out of balance and there is a potential for illness. Reiki restores natural balance and supports the body's ability to heal itself. It is used to treat a variety of physical ailments, such as headaches, migraines, sinus problems, frequent colds, flu, coughs, back pain, cystitis, stomach ache, infections, kidney and gallbladder stones, aches and pains in the joints (see Chapter 7, page 156). For a sick person, Reiki can support resumption of complete physical health or can limit the symptoms. Reiki energy helps many conditions, both acute and chronic, and always contributes towards healing. Chronic ailments often take longer to heal and need Reiki to be applied more often.

On the emotional level

Reiki has a relaxing, calming effect on the nervous system and brings balance to uneven emotions. While receiving a Reiki treatment or taking part in Reiki training, your emotions may be profoundly affected. Emotional blockages can be released, and as a consequence tears may flow or the laughter of relief may come spontaneously. Reiki helps us become more aware of our inner emotional processes. We come into closer contact with suppressed feelings: sadness, fear or anger. These 'negative' energies need to be acknowledged before they can be transformed into their positive opposites: joy, courage and compassion. Without exposing these energies and giving them the attention and expression they need, we cannot let go of them and use them as a creative force.

Reiki energy balances and harmonizes, and is very useful in cases of shock (physical and emotional) and after accidents (see page 161). Today stress is a common experience in daily life; we need to learn to replenish our energy in order to keep stress levels to a minimum, and Reiki can help us do this, since its energy allows us to let go and relax. At the same time it can influence and change mental attitudes by suggesting new perspectives and positive reactions to stressful situations.

On the mental level

Reiki works by relaxing and calming the mind's activity. This enables the receiver to gain enhanced clarity, perhaps about a current life issue or by becoming aware of inner processes, such as a negative self-belief. During a Reiki treatment it is not unusual for the receiver to experience insights that provide clarity on decisions to bring about changes and improve life.

On the spiritual level

Receiving and giving Reiki reconnects us to the Source and to unconditional love. It invites us to think and feel 'wider' and 'bigger'. It enhances our awareness and puts us in touch with our true Divine essence. After a Reiki treatment, receivers often feel that they are in contact with something more profound than their usual self – as though they have entered a deeper level, where they connect with their inner being.

Reiki works on the body as a whole, balancing the emotions, bringing clarity to the mind and reconnecting to the 'true' self, which in turn impacts on physical well-being.

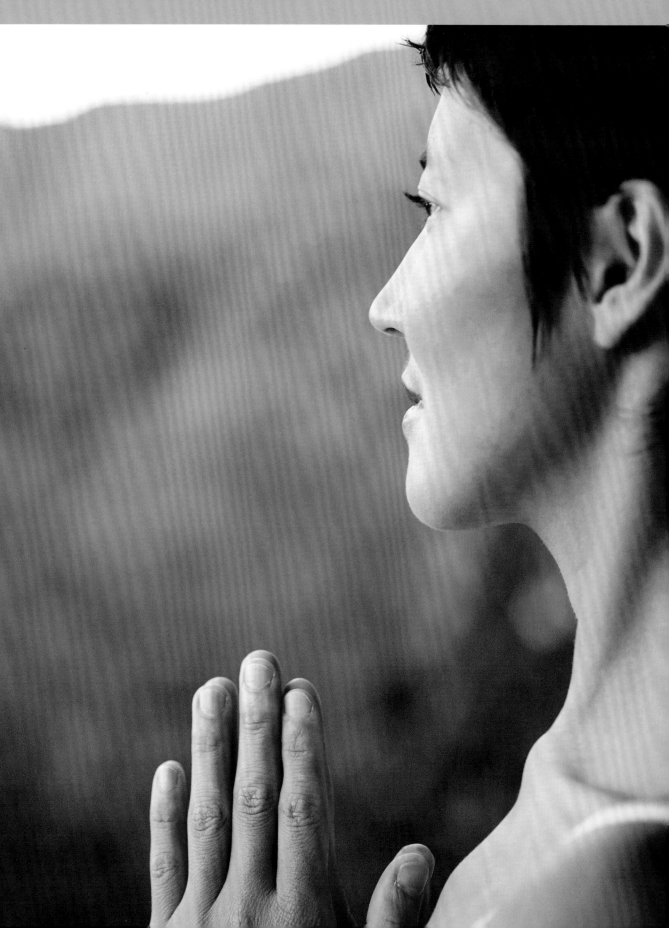

Channels and channelling

A channel is a metaphysical conduit through which energy can pass, and we can talk about a person becoming a 'channel' for this energy. Someone who has trained in Reiki has become a channel for Reiki energy, enabling them to pass it on to others.

Access to the Higher Self

The more we allow ourselves to be used as a channel for Reiki, the more Reiki spreads through our life, enriching every aspect of it. The empowerment given through attunement is like opening an existing channel within, connecting us to our Higher Self, Soul or Spirit, which is in turn connected to the Source, to Divine essence, to God. The Higher Self represents our superconscious level (see page 85). It is our 'true' self; alert and full of light, it can see things clearly. For example, it knows our true purpose in life and the experiences we have chosen in order to learn certain lessons. This part is guiding us, providing us with intuition and insight, always loving and supporting us for our highest and greatest good.

Contacting Reiki energy

In a Reiki treatment, the giver is used as a channel to conduct Universal Life Energy to the receiver. The moment you are attuned to Reiki energy in First Degree training (see page 66), you are able to access this energy to heal yourself and others. The 'success' of an attunement does not depend on you, since no special preparation, knowledge or skills are needed to become a Reiki channel. The Reiki energy flows from an inexhaustible universal source and reconnects you with your own ability to access it. Each attunement, as you work through the three Reiki degrees, increasingly opens up your own inner healing channel. The more often you act as a channel, the more easily and strongly the energy flows through it. Even if you do not practise Reiki for a while, you never lose this ability, though after a long break you might need to disperse blockages. Imagine a pipe that is used regularly, through which water runs clear and clean; if this pipe is used only occasionally, contaminants can accumulate and impede the flow.

Opening up your intuition

Practising Reiki opens up your intuition. After a time you start to trust yourself more, knowing exactly where to place your hands on the receiver's body, where your hands are most needed. Intuition is part of our Higher Intelligence and is connected to our Higher Self. From this level we receive inner guidance. We can ask any question and we will receive the answer. We are all aware of situations in our lives when we know intuitively, from a gut feeling, what it feels right to do, even though the logical mind may be sceptical. Later we realize that our intuitive decision was right, and we feel released, having trusted it. In the physical body, intuition is connected with the right side of the brain and the left side of the body.

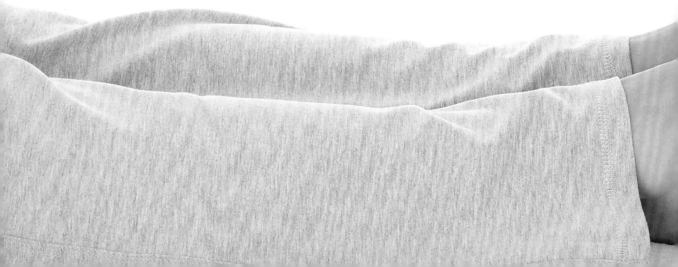

Once you have trained in Reiki, you will become a channel for its healing energy, and the more you practise Reiki, the wider the channel becomes and the more powerful the energy flow.

People who rely on creativity in their work often say that the inspiration for a new task came 'out of the blue', when they were completely relaxed; suddenly a solution presented itself to them. Einstein, Edison and Archimedes all found the last piece of the puzzle in their world-changing discoveries in a deeply relaxed state of body and mind. In important decisions and dilemmas we are guided by our Higher Intelligence, when our logical mind is still and intuition can lead us.

Wisdom and language of the body

Our body has its own wisdom, sending us signals and relaying messages. From a holistic viewpoint, any disease has a reason that underlies the presenting symptom. If we treat only the symptom, the illness might abate, but it will eventually return if the root cause is not dealt with. There are also other points to consider.

Finding the underlying cause

Each disease is a result of an imbalance in life. Reiki can help find the underlying cause of the illness (the imbalance), as it always works on the person as a 'whole', integrating all levels of the body: the mind, the emotions and the spirit.

As a Reiki healer, it is helpful to encourage a receiver to look at their lifestyle and at any life issues that may need changing for the 'highest good'. Because Reiki works on emotional, mental and spiritual levels, the cause is treated as well as the illness.

The body as a temple

Although it may be a modern-day cliché, from a spiritual viewpoint the body is indeed a 'temple', providing us with shelter and housing. We can also look on the body as a friend who always wants to help and support us, keeping us healthy and happy. If something goes 'wrong' or is not moving in the direction that life wants us to progress in, either in our thinking or in more general ways, we then receive signals from the body – in other words, a message from our friend.

The body is trying to tell us something when we experience pain, infection or a physical symptom. We may not understand this message, and the usual reaction is to try to get rid of the physical symptom as quickly as possible. However, if we really want the body to be properly healed – and not just the symptom dealt with – we need to listen to the body and understand the underlying cause. When we are willing, by sensitively listening to the signals that the body produces, we can pick up messages in the 'energy body' (see page 34) before an imbalance manifests itself in physical form as a disease or illness.

QUESTIONS TO ASK

The following questions can help you work out what the underlying cause of an illness might be:

- What am I ignoring in my life?
- What is trying to attract my attention?
- What does this disease, pain or infection seem to be communicating?
- What does the sick part of the body need from me?
- What do I need to be aware of and learn?
- What do I need to do to become completely healthy and whole again?
- What should I do to love, accept and heal myself?

'Reiki helps people to attain an inner peace and inner knowing of themselves so that they don't have to rely on others for healing.'

Bernard

In order to truly understand and combat physical illness, we need to tune into the body's signals and messages, which can warn us of potential health problems.

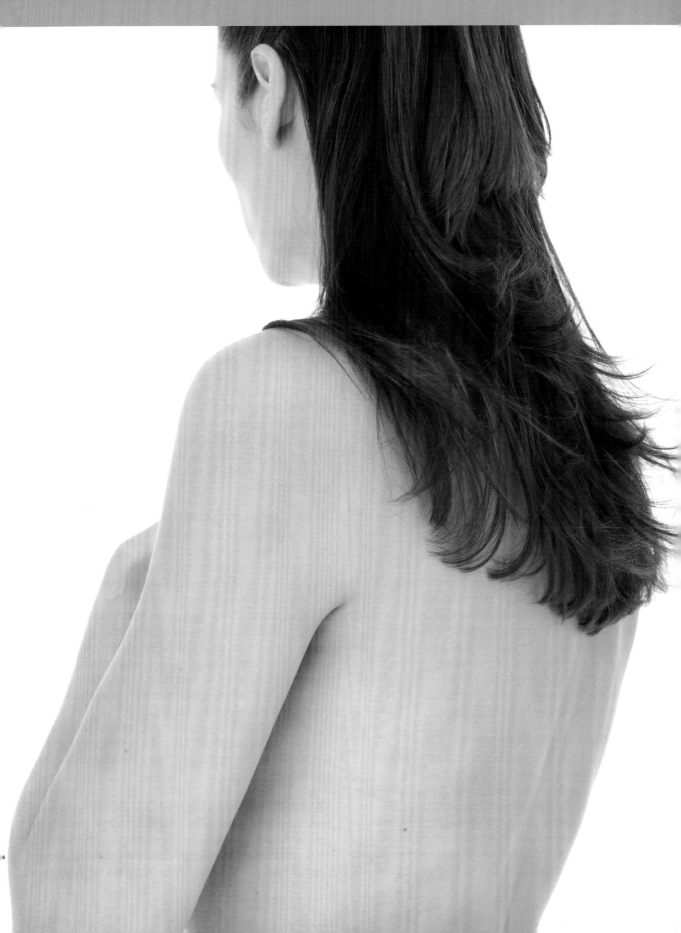

The chakras and the endocrine system

Chakra is a Sanskrit word meaning 'wheel' or 'vortex'. The chakras are vital energy centres, relating to the energy bodies of the human aura. Each chakra is connected to one of the seven energy bodies. For example, the first energy body (etheric) is associated with the first chakra, the second body (emotional) with the second chakra, and so on (see page 34).

Major and minor chakras

There are seven major chakras located in the seven main energy bodies. In addition, there are more than 20 minor chakras, such as those in the palms of each hand and on the knees and soles of the feet. A healthy chakra vibrates evenly in a circular motion; it resembles a funnel, becoming wider as it gets further away from the body. The chakras are vortices that govern our physical, emotional, mental and spiritual well-being.

Healthy and unhealthy chakras

When a chakra is healthy, balanced and open, those specific parts of the body linked with it are healthy, too. When a chakra is blocked, damaged or closed, the balance in the chakra is disturbed and this is reflected in the health of the connected part of the physical body. Our chakras are affected by everything that happens to us. If good things occur – for example, we fall in love – we feel light and sparkling and have lots of energy. The opposite happens when we feel 'under the weather', emotionally depressed or in a bad mood, and this can have a harmful effect on our energy system.

When energy is held back from its natural flow – for instance, when we suppress a feeling or stifle actions because of fear – the body can create a protective barrier in the form and texture of our tissue (as dense, hard or tense tissue). A good body therapist can tell, by looking at the physical structure of muscles, bones and tissue, where unexpressed energies are contained. This does not necessarily result in disease, but represents a limitation of expression through the physical body and can cause discomfort in related areas.

Each chakra reflects an aspect of our personal growth. A disturbance in the first chakra (root or base chakra)

might manifest as a problem in finding a job and making money. This lesson has to do with 'standing on our own feet'. Energy has to be constantly flowing through our system in order for us to remain in optimum health. An imbalance of energy or a blockage in the chakras can cause illness.

The body's endocrine system

You can integrate the harmonizing of each chakra into a single Reiki treatment. The basic Reiki hand positions follow the location of the seven main chakras and correspond with the body's endocrine glandular system (see panel opposite). The endocrine system regulates balance of the hormones and the metabolism. On an energetic level, the endocrine glands correspond to the seven main chakras.

The hormones produced by the ductless glands of the endocrine system flow directly into the bloodstream or the circulation, bringing vital energy into the body, either to stimulate or hinder the activity of other organs and tissues. Hormones are produced in minute quantities, but their effects are profound: some are long-lasting, others only temporary. The endocrine system provides power to the chakras and, at the same time, leads their subtle energies (energies that are charged with a higher vibration and that permeate and envelop the physical body) back into the body. Reiki healing operates through interaction between the chakras and the endocrine glands.

Usui and Takata always emphasized the importance of the harmony of the endocrine system and of balancing the chakras. Any overactivity or underactivity of one gland affects the entire system. Our hormones regulate the vital processes of the body, such as metabolism,

THE MAIN ENDOCRINE GLANDS

Each gland influences the production of particular hormones:

- The pineal gland secretes a hormone that may help regulate patterns of sleeping and waking.
- The pituitary gland, often called the 'master gland', produces hormones that control several other endocrine glands.
- The thyroid (and parathyroid) gland hormones control the rate at which cells burn fuel from food in order to produce energy.
- The thymus gland plays an important part in the development of the immune system in early life.
- The adrenal glands play a large role in regulating the body's response to stress, balancing the immune system and metabolism.
- The gonads (testes in men and ovaries in women) secrete the sex hormones testosterone in men and oestrogen and progesterone in women, which control sexual development, sex drive and fertility.
- The islets of Langerhans, specialized cells in the pancreas, function as endocrine glands. They secrete the insulin needed for the metabolism of sugar.

The hormones secreted by each of these endocrine glands have a dramatic effect on human psychology, and imbalances in them can cause both physical and emotional problems.

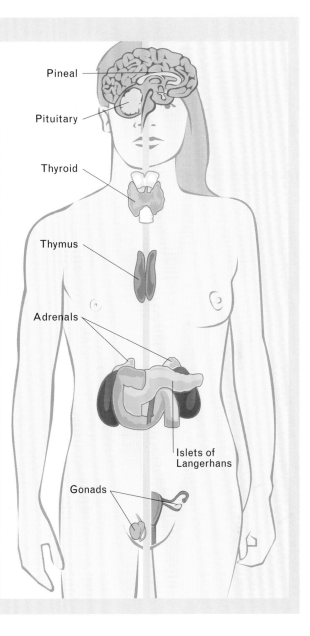

Pineal
Pituitary
Thyroid
Thymus
Adrenals
Islets of Langerhans
Gonads

growth, ageing, resistance to stress, the body's ability to heal itself and reproduction.

The endocrine system works together with the autonomous nervous system to control the internal environment of the body and acts as part of its communication system. Stress is one of the major causes when the balance of the body's metabolism is disturbed. The basic Reiki hand positions (see pages 128–140) align with the location of the endocrine glands. Full body treatments with Reiki reduce tension and stress and support the body's natural ability to heal itself.

'Reiki healing operates through interaction between the chakras and the endocrine glands.'

Qualities and functions of the seven main chakras

All the chakras (except the crown chakra) are linked to certain parts of the body. When the energy of one chakra is not in balance, disturbances in the connected parts of the body can occur. For example, an imbalance in the root chakra is connected with the hands and feet, and reflects our security in the world.

What are the chakras for?

Each chakra is linked with a specific organ and area of the body, and has an influence on its function. The chakras open to both the front and the back of the body. The front aspects of the chakras are concerned with the emotions, and the back aspects with the person's will. All chakras are openings enabling energy to flow in and out of the aura, as well as into and out of the physical body. Each chakra absorbs Universal Energy (*ki, chi* or *prana*), breaks it up into component parts and then sends it along energy lines (nadis) to the nervous system, the endocrine glands and the blood, to nourish the body.

'The chakras are vortices that govern our physical, emotional, mental and spiritual well-being.'

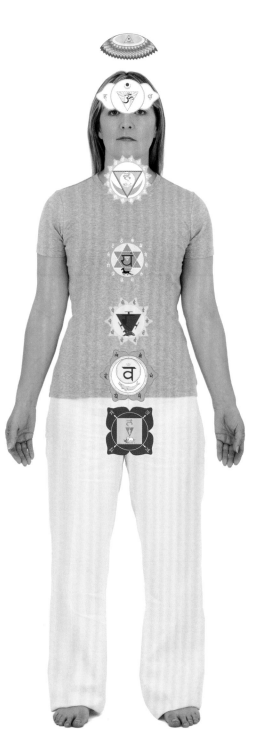

The seven main chakras on the body range from the root (first) chakra in the pubic-bone area to the crown (seventh) chakra at the top of the head.

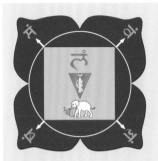

THE ROOT OR FIRST CHAKRA (MULADHARA)

Location	Base of the spine, where the sacrum joins the coccyx (on the back of the body); pubic-bone area (on the front of the body)
Linked with	Feet and legs
Colours	Red and yellow
Element	Earth
Body parts/organs	Adrenal glands, bladder, genitals, spine, hips
Functions	Creative expression, abundance, seat of Kundalini energy (strong energy that normally rests like a serpent at the base of the spine, but can be awakened through meditation)
Associated life themes	Will to live, survival, power, aggression, security, grounding, money, job, fertility, home, sense of belonging, confidence, 'fight or flight' response, self-acceptance

Possible problems when the chakra is not in balance

Emotional	Fear of being in the world, feeling threatened in the above areas, aggressiveness, defensive attitude, unreliability, jumpiness, tendency to panic attacks
Physical	Digestive disorders: chronic diarrhoea, enteritis, constipation, haemorrhoids, impotence; problems with: anus, large intestine, coccyx, sacrum, spine, lower back

Imbalances

When underactive	Insecure, passive, suppressed, finding it difficult to say 'no', prone to panic, tearful, withdrawn, not present, likely to be 'wavering'
When overactive	Very aggressive, proud, finding it difficult to say 'yes', inflexible, dogmatic
In balance	True to yourself, steady, unshaken

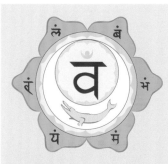

THE SACRAL OR SECOND CHAKRA (SVADHISTHANA)

Location	Between the pubic bone and the navel (about 5 cm/2 in below the navel)
Linked with	Ankles and wrists
Colours	Orange and red
Element	Water
Body parts/organs	Reproductive organs, testes (in men), ovaries (in women), fluid functions of the body, digestive organs, kidneys, urinary tract, lower back
Functions	Feelings, emotional centre and the focus of sexual and sensual energies
Associated life themes	Vitality, enjoyment of life, sexuality, sensuality, refinement of feelings, relationships, sharing, intimacy, pleasure, sensations, appetite, desires, self-esteem

Possible problems when the chakra is not in balance

Emotional	Lack of self-love and self-acceptance, problems with themes in the above areas, difficulty in digesting the emotions, inability to commit, no sexual satisfaction (frigidity, impotence and premature ejaculation)
Physical	Problems with: genitals, prostate glands, reproductive organs, large and small intestine, bladder, appendix, stomach, sciatic nerve, lower back, sacrum, lumbar region

Imbalances

When underactive	Feeling guilty, with low self-esteem, fearful of being punished or repressed
When overactive	Addicted to pleasure, lustful, using others for sexual pleasure
In balance	Open, receiving, enjoying having fun

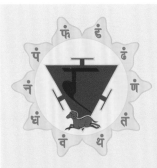

THE SOLAR-PLEXUS OR THIRD CHAKRA (MANIPURA)

Location	At the solar plexus, between the navel and base of the ribcage
Linked with	Lower legs and lower arms
Colours	Yellow and red
Element	Fire
Body parts/organs	Stomach, liver, adrenals, gallbladder, pancreas, solar plexus, spleen, digestive system, middle back
Functions	Power and wisdom centre
Associated life themes	Personal power, dominance, will, control, self-determination, strength, self-empowerment, purpose, fear or anxiety, weakness

Possible problems when the chakra is not in balance

Emotional	Feeling of being blocked, guilt and shame, rationalization of feelings, dependency in relationships
Physical	Problems with: the above organs, duodenum, lymphatic system, kidneys, lumbar region; repressed energy at cell level may lead to cancer, arthritis, anorexia, bulimia, ulcers

Imbalances

When underactive	Passive, weak, emotionally repressed and withdrawn, with a strong connection and attachment to people and things, drawing in energy, intimidated, obedient, finding it difficult to relate to people
When overactive	Overreacting, liking dramas, manipulative, dominant, tyrannical, overbearing, suffering from low self-esteem, competitive, controlling of others, undermining others
In balance	Spontaneous, detached from people and things, having a healthy self-esteem, self-controlling, effective in the world

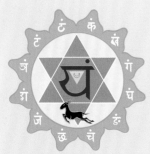

THE HEART OR FOURTH CHAKRA (ANAHATA)

Location	Middle of the chest
Linked with	Knees, elbows, pelvis area
Colours	Green and pink
Element	Air
Body parts/organs	Heart, thymus gland, lungs, circulation and blood pressure, immune system, upper back, arms, hands
Functions	Love, compassion
Associated life themes	Being able to give and receive love, unconditional love, unity, compassion, kindness, self-love, peace, trust, spiritual development, forgiveness

Possible problems when the chakra is not in balance

Emotional	Fear of love and intimacy, fear of being touched physically, fear of letting others in, potentially psychopathic
Physical	Problems with: the heart, heart attacks, blood pressure and circulation, diseases of the immune system and thymus gland, arteries, breasts, hips, lungs, bronchia, oesophagus, diaphragm, thoracic spine

Imbalances

When underactive	Fearful of love, unwilling to give love, pragmatic and egoistic when there is weakness in the heart, lost in emotions, misunderstandings and disputes
When overactive	(Not applicable)
In balance	Showing impersonal feelings and unconditional love, empathizing, responsible, full of goodwill, compassionate, devoted and humble, open-minded and outgoing, giving selflessly without any expectations

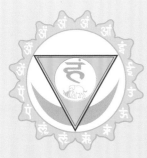

THE THROAT OR FIFTH CHAKRA (VISHUDHA)

Location	Throat area
Linked with	Pelvis area and shoulders
Colours	Blue
Element	Ether
Body parts/organs	Throat, voice, thyroid gland, upper lungs and arms, digestive tract, neck, lower jaw, oesophagus, metabolism
Functions	Communication
Associated life themes	Self-expression, communication, being able to receive and accept love and devotion, creativity, sense of responsibility, abundance

Possible problems when the chakra is not in balance

Emotional	Rigidity, unwillingness to compromise, frustration in communication, fear of expressing yourself and developing your own individuality
Physical	Problems with: throat, neck, shoulders, thyroid, thymus gland, lungs, immune system, bronchia, nervous system, mouth, teeth, tongue, jawbone, trachea, cervical spine

Imbalances

When underactive	Unable to communicate (swallowing what you want to say), missing creative and verbal expression, lacking devotion
When overactive	Excessively interested in worldly things, overly impartial (objective)
In balance	Able to develop and grow in your own creative expression, able to say what you need to say, having a good self-image and inner acceptance, devoted, trustworthy and peaceful; singing (and perhaps painting) helps to balance the throat chakra

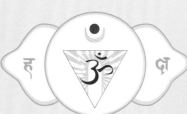

THE THIRD-EYE OR SIXTH CHAKRA (AJNA)

Location	Between the eyebrows, about 2.5 cm (1 in) above the centre of the eyebrows
Linked with	Forehead
Colours	Indigo and moonstone
Element	(None)
Body parts/organs	Pituitary gland, lower brain, hypothalamus, eyes, nose, spine, ears, autonomic nervous system
Functions	Intuitive centre, seat of will and clairvoyance
Associated life themes	Thought control, inner vision and understanding, telepathy, inspiration, spiritual awakening, imagination, insights, integrated personality

Possible problems when the chakra is not in balance

Emotional	Feeling rational and judgemental, illusions, hallucinations, hiding feelings behind thoughts
Physical	Brain tumours, strokes, insomnia, hormonal imbalances, headaches, migraines, sinusitis, dizziness, depression; diseases of the autonomous nervous system, the ears, eyes, spine and endocrine system; problems with: the left hemisphere of the brain and the right eye

Imbalances

When underactive	Identity-less, confused
When overactive	Controlling, ambitious, having a strong ego and programmed actions, disrespectful of others
In balance	Experiencing Divine joy, spiritual awareness, god-consciousness and joyful configuration; meditation helps to open the third-eye chakra

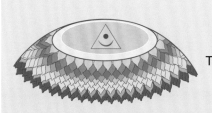

THE CROWN OR SEVENTH CHAKRA (SAHASRARA)

The crown chakra is the highest chakra and cannot be influenced in terms of opening or closing. It opens automatically when we develop spiritually. When we are spiritually awake, this chakra is open and there is cosmic consciousness, unity with the Divine and with all things; we are aliveness, joy, acceptance and playfulness.

Location	On the top (crown) of the head
Linked with	Pineal gland
Colours	Violet (purple) and white
Element	(None)
Body parts/organs	Pineal gland, upper brain, nervous system
Function	Connection to the Higher Self
Associated life themes	Consciousness of oneness, self-realization, spiritual awareness, wisdom, extended consciousness, intuition, connection to the Higher Self, to the inner guidance and to all-embracing love, completion
Possible problems	When the chakra is not developed, someone is too materialistic (clinging to the material plane)
Possible diseases	Disturbances in brain function and the nerves, tumours, strokes, problems with the spine; serious psychotic disorders, being totally cut off, in deep shock, inability to face up to reality

Balancing chakra energy

To maintain your physical, emotional, mental and spiritual health, it is important to arrive at a balance between the energies of your chakras. Each one reflects special qualities, functions and aspects of personal growth.

Imbalance in the chakras

When someone pays too much attention to one chakra, this can lead to physical disorders and illnesses. For example, too much attention to the second chakra can manifest as an addiction to pleasure – perhaps to excessive sex, eating or drinking too much alcohol or even taking drugs. You can balance these energies by carrying out Reiki on the throat (fifth) and sacral (second) chakras. Through creative self-expression and activities such as singing, writing or painting, this attachment can be dissolved. Someone who has a physical problem in one part of the body often carries an imbalance (or physical problem) in the area of the corresponding chakra. For instance, someone with constant problems in the throat area may also have physical problems in the lower back or with the reproductive organs, which correspond with the second chakra. By laying on hands and giving Reiki to the throat area and lower back (treating from the front), you can balance and harmonize the energies in those two chakras (second and fifth chakras). The seventh chakra is the highest chakra and is different from all the others; it does not need to be influenced or balanced. We do not touch it, as it does not need additional energy.

When there is too much energy in the head and too little in the lower body, leave one hand resting on the forehead (sixth chakra) and lay the other hand on all the chakras, one after the other, starting with the first chakra. This way the energy gets drawn from the head area into the lower part of the body. The same applies to the first chakra. Lay one hand on the first chakra and balance all the other chakras with it, one after the other. Balancing the sixth chakra with the second chakra has a deeply relaxing effect, too.

HARMONIZING THE CHAKRAS

To achieve a good balance, it is important that each chakra harmonizes with the one directly above it. It is also fundamental that the three lower chakras harmonize with the three higher ones. The energy of the first chakra (survival, security, confidence) needs to harmonize with the energy of the fourth chakra (love, trust, compassion). The energy of the second chakra (enjoyment, sensuality, desire) needs to be balanced with the energy of the fifth chakra (expression, creativity, devotion), and the third chakra (power, ego-will, dominance) with the energy of the sixth chakra (inner vision, God's will, understanding).

first, root chakra >> fourth, heart chakra
second, sacral chakra >> fifth, throat chakra
third, solar-plexus chakra >> sixth, third-eye chakra

BALANCING THE CHAKRAS IN TURN

A simple way to keep all your chakras balanced is shown in the following sequence of treatment positions, in which you can balance the chakras in turn. Let your hands rest on the two chakras until you feel the same energy in both of them. You may feel a temperature difference at the two points, ranging from warm to cold; wait until you feel both hands become equally warm. This can take 2–5 minutes.

first, root chakra >> sixth, third-eye chakra
second, sacral chakra >> fifth, throat chakra
third, solar-plexus chakra >> fourth, heart chakra

Self-balancing the chakras

This form of Reiki treatment helps you revitalize and balance your chakras, to enable your energy to flow freely and keep you healthy. Let your hands rest for about three to five minutes in each specified position.

Instructions

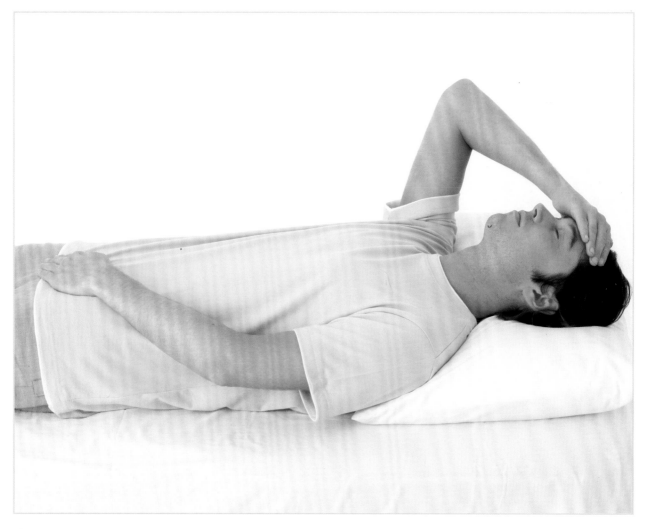

1 Place one hand on your sixth chakra (your forehead) and the other over the first chakra (pubic-bone area). This balances the energy of the head and lower parts of the body. We often have too much energy in the head and too little in the lower abdomen. This puts you more in touch with your sexual energy.

2 Lay one hand over your fifth chakra (throat) and the other on your second chakra (below the navel). This balances the emotions and vitality with the area of self-expression and communication. You will feel more connected with your emotions and desires and be able to express them more easily, in a creative way.

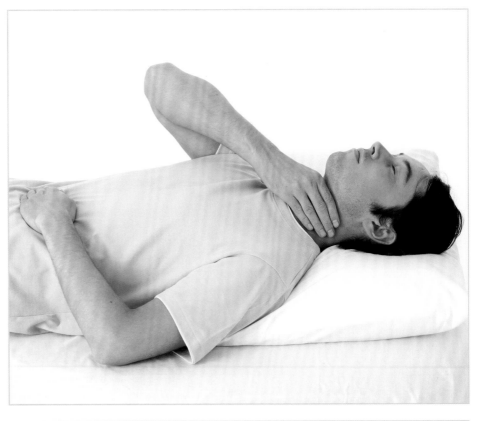

3 Lay one hand on the fourth chakra (middle of the chest) and the other on the third chakra (solar plexus). The heart stands for love and compassion and the solar plexus for your personal strength and power. If these centres are balanced, the right decisions are made through love and understanding.

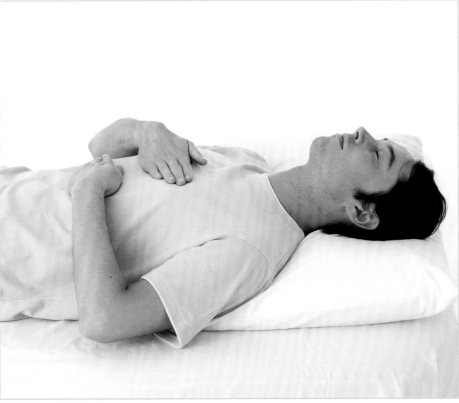

4 Place one hand on your second chakra (below the navel) and the other on the sixth chakra (forehead). This position relaxes you deeply and allows you to let go of thoughts and feelings.

5 After you have balanced all your chakras, move your body gently, wiggle your toes and fingers and stretch your whole body. Come back to normal consciousness.

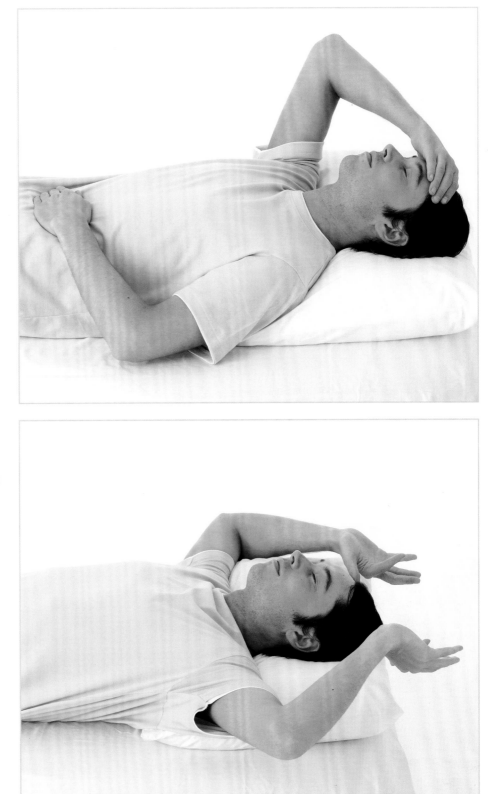

After-effects of Reiki

The most important effect Reiki has is on the mental and spiritual level, because our mental forces are very powerful. Reiki enhances spiritual growth, and Reiki initiates gain greater clarity about themselves and their lives. They feel as if their consciousness has expanded and this often leads to personal insights, in turn bringing positive life changes. They feel strength and courage, and are charged with energy to make the right decisions and to accomplish what is best for themselves and others.

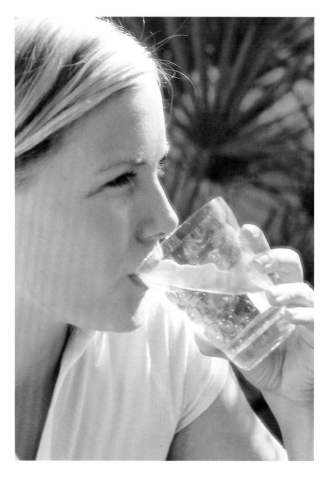

To aid the deep-cleansing process that Reiki treatment or attunement to Reiki energy prompts, make sure that you drink plenty of water (see page 52).

The healing and cleansing process

Reiki can heal difficult relationships and often brings people closer together; it supports spiritual growth whenever we allow it to. Reiki always works for our 'highest best and good' and encompasses changes in our lives – for example, changes in relationships, at work, at home or in any particular situation.

A deep cleansing happens whenever we receive Reiki treatment or are being attuned to Reiki energy (see also pages 71 and 76). On the physical level, Reiki cleanses the body of toxins and supports the healing process. To help the cleansing process on the physical level, it is recommended that you drink lots of water after attunement and Reiki treatment.

Cleansing effects

On an emotional level, Reiki loosens blocked energy that has been trapped in the muscles, tissues, organs and even the bones. This energy can shift and be released, in order to flow freely again. In the beginning this may be unpleasant for the receiver (see page 71), but after attunement, many Reiki initiates experience a deep emotional and spiritual encounter with themselves. A space of peace, quiet and meditation opens up, which engulfs the Reiki Master and student together. After each Reiki degree and after each attunement, many positive changes take place for students. Many of them relate how they feel more at peace, less fearful and more patient, and they sleep better, feel more positive and have more energy in general. Often students feel their body temperature rising, especially in their hands, as if something is burning within them.

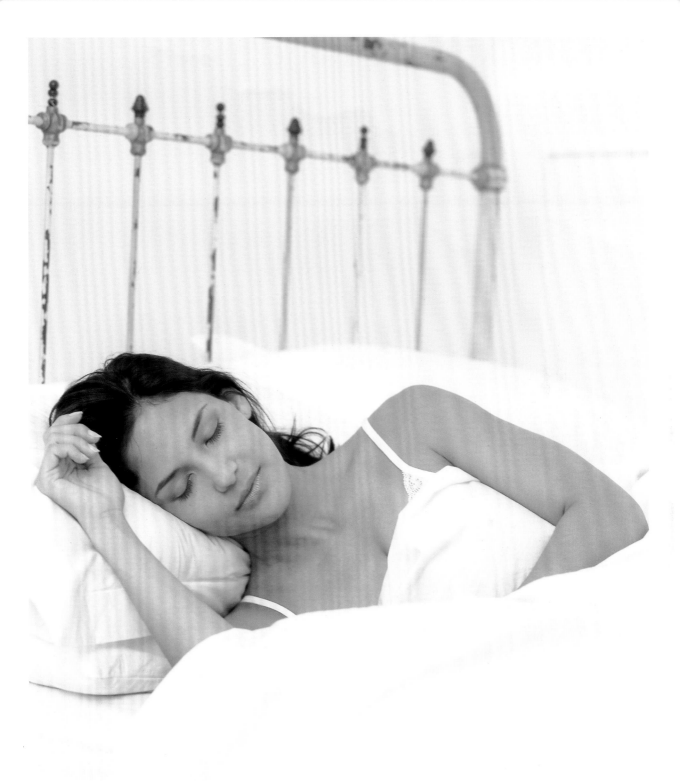

Many Reiki students experience several positive emotional and physical effects following each attunement, including a profound sense of peace and the ability to sleep soundly.

How Reiki knowledge builds

Reiki is usually taught at three main levels or degrees (First, Second and Third). At each level you receive one or more attunements. With each degree you become a wider channel through which Reiki healing energy can flow. Each energy-transmission (initiation) expands your Reiki channel and increases the amount of Reiki flowing through you.

Receiving attunements

In the First Degree you receive four attunements over two days so that your body can slowly open to the higher vibration of energy, which builds up with each attunement. In the Second Degree the attunement is single and very powerful, because you receive the empowerment of the three Reiki symbols. Sometimes this can stimulate strong healing reactions in the physical body, such as fever or the feeling of impending illness. These reactions usually last only a short time, and may occur overnight and be gone the next morning. In the Third Degree initiates receive a single attunement that broadens the healing channel and deepens meditation (see page 114).

What is an attunement?

In Reiki, attunement means 'initiation' or 'to get attuned to' becoming a channel for Universal Life Energy. You receive an attunement to the Reiki power (also called 'energy-transmission' or 'initiation'). Using an ancient technique, the Reiki Master transmits energy to the student. The attunement process usually takes the form of a simple ceremony in which the Reiki Master uses the confidential Reiki symbols and mantras. Each energy transmission opens up the inner healing channel and amplifies the flow of energy. The energy enters the body through the top of the head and flows through the upper energy centres (chakras). It continues down the arms and leaves the body via the hands.

Attunement is the special key to the Reiki system and makes it a unique healing method, quite different from other hands-on techniques. Usui discovered the symbols and mantras in sacred Sanskrit scriptures, but was unable to use them for healing until he was empowered through his enlightened experience at Mount Kurama (see page 12). Without the attunement, which is a transmission of energy, the symbols do not activate the Reiki energy.

Initiation into Reiki creates an ongoing channel in your energy body through which Reiki flows. At the end of the attunements of each degree, the Master 'seals' the channel. From now on you have your own direct connection to channel Reiki energy.

The effects of attunement

The major effect of an attunement is that is clears and cleanses the whole energy body, as each attunement raises the vibratory level at which we normally function. This results in a 21-day cleansing process by the Reiki energy (see page 76). It is good to support this process by giving yourself a full Reiki treatment daily (or at least half an hour), and to drink more water than you usually do (2–3 litres/3½–5 pints a day).

'The Reiki First Degree gave me a great confidence, and a place in the world I had not known before. It empowered me. The Second Degree reveals to me that there has been a deep and serious imbalance in my life, which has always been with me. It shows the need and gives me the tools to put things right.'

Sarah

In the Second Degree attunement, in a single intense process the Reiki Master uses the Reiki symbols and corresponding mantras to amplify the flow of energy to the initiate (see page 79).

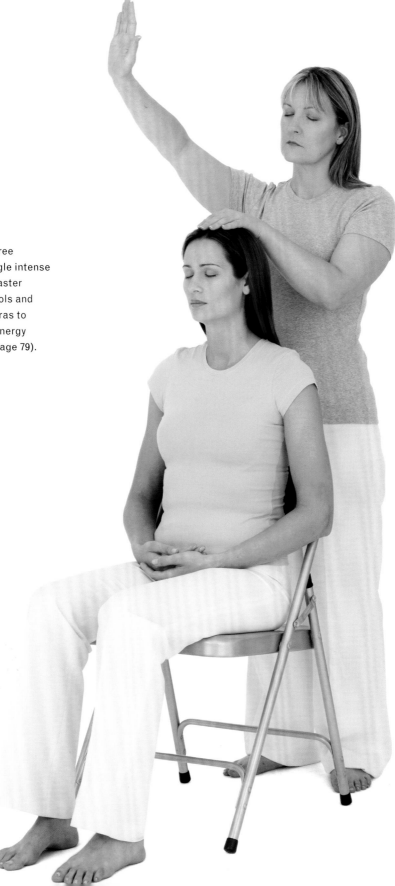

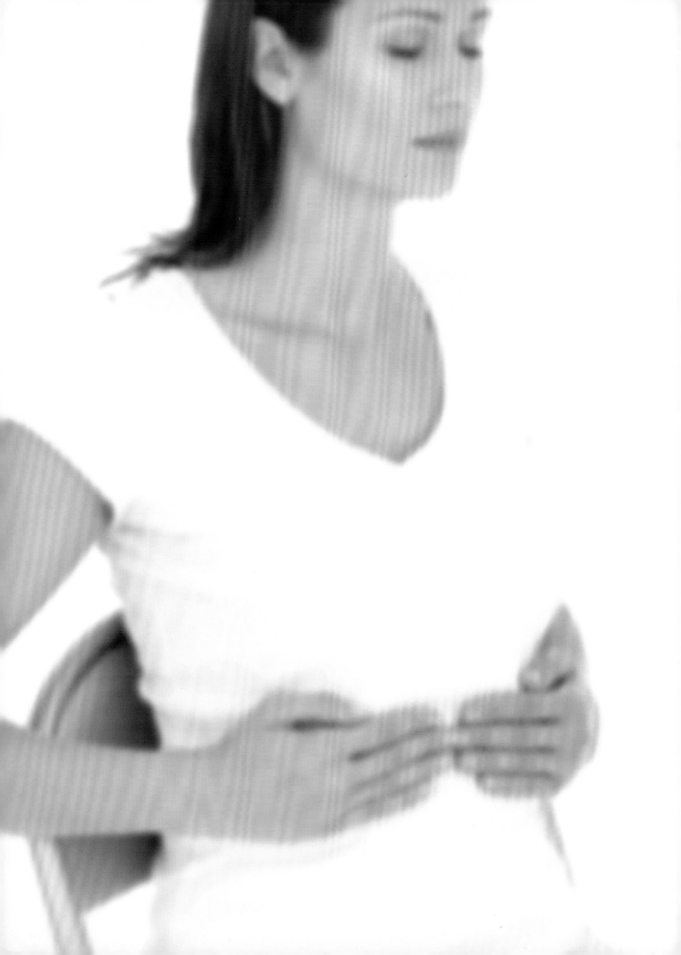

The First Degree

Reiki is a healing method that you do not need any prior experience or special skills to learn. Everyone can practise Reiki, irrespective of age, creed or knowledge, and can use Reiki on themselves initially, and then to heal others. The only prerequisite is to be receptive and open to letting this healing power flow through you. The first step in becoming a Reiki healer is to take the First Degree. This teaches you the essential hand positions, equipping you to carry out self-healing as well as healing on family and friends.

What you learn in the First Degree

The First Degree training is a basic course held over two days or four consecutive evenings. Each session lasts about three hours, during which you receive the four attunements and are taught the fundamentals of the Reiki system of healing, its history, effects and benefits. Furthermore you learn and practise the basic hand positions in order to treat yourself and others. You also learn some additional hand positions, how to treat animals and how to use Reiki in first aid.

The emphasis of the First Degree

The techniques learnt in the First Degree are complete in themselves. If you feel drawn to work with the Reiki energy at a deeper level, then the Second Degree training is recommended. There should be a minimum period of 2–3 months' practice with Reiki at the First Degree to adjust your energy to the higher vibration frequency and to gain sufficient experience and confidence before moving on to a higher level.

A major part of the Reiki method is the emphasis on self-treatment; healing yourself is a strong focus in the First Degree. Reiki naturally opens the door for people to become loving and caring towards themselves; before we can 'help' or 'heal' others, we have to start with ourselves. We can only give to others what we are prepared to give to ourselves. This means taking responsibility for our own healing, health and well-being. Because Reiki is a gentle and non-intrusive technique, beginners need not be nervous of trying it out. Laying hands on your own body becomes an expression and acknowledgement of being loving to yourself. Giving a Reiki self-treatment becomes an important part of your life (see pages 128–132 for the self-treatment hand positions).

Daily self-treatment

After the First Degree, it is a good idea to work on yourself every day. This strengthens your health, and your life-force energy is recharged with each session. Using Reiki regularly may bring up things that have been held back or stored beneath the surface, especially at emotional and mental levels. When energy begins to shift and blockages are slowly removed, the process is not always a smooth one. It will require your conscious effort and a readiness to look at emotions and situations, so that you can learn from them and perhaps change things in your life for the better.

Facing negativity

When negative unconscious beliefs, thoughts, emotions and attitudes towards ourselves and our lives start surfacing, we are challenged and may need to confront old problems from long ago. This is a necessary part of healing on a deeper level. Whatever needs to be healed has first to surface and expose itself to the open, like a wound that requires sun and air in order to heal. It is important to persevere and to understand that this is part of the healing process. It can sometimes take weeks, months or even years. When we accept and support this process, we benefit and gradually feel better than ever before. We become more vital and lighter, in contact with our own energy and feelings, and generally happier, healthier and more contented.

The First Degree primarily focuses on self-treatment, where you learn the basic hand positions, such as Head Position Two shown here, which harmonizes the two sides of the brain.

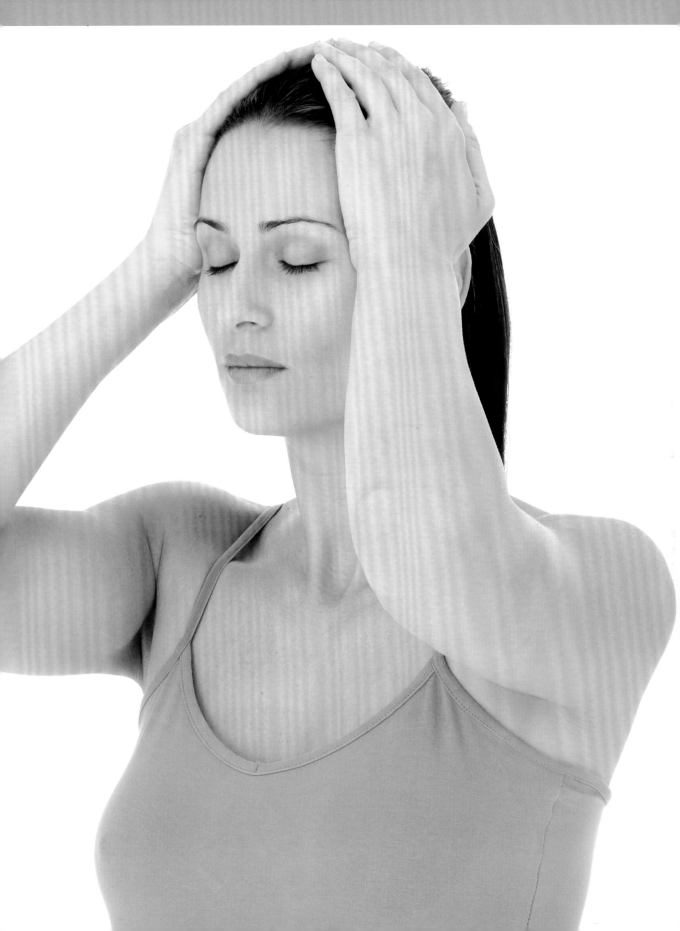

Preparing to treat others

No special preparation is needed to treat yourself or others with Reiki. You just need to place your hands on those parts of the body that require relaxation or healing. If you come across a chronic problem or disease, such as migraines, a lower-back problem or a digestive complaint, you should work with Reiki full treatments over a period of time (see pages 128–140 for all the relevant hand positions). Additionally, you may want to consult a medical practitioner.

Centring yourself

At the start of the treatment you need to centre yourself. Spend a few moments breathing deeply and begin relaxing your body. In addition, place your hands on the second chakra (below the navel, see page 67). Relax into this area while breathing, becoming aware of the rise and fall of your belly, and connect with this centre for a few moments. Another way to centre yourself is in the fourth chakra (heart centre, see page 61). Place both hands on the centre of your chest, relax your breathing and connect with your heart and a feeling of love and peace within.

Treatment surfaces

To make practical preparations for giving a Reiki treatment, you need to establish a quiet, safe and comfortable environment. Take whatever steps are necessary to ensure that you are not going to be disturbed during the period of the treatment. Set up a treatment table – a massage table is perfect. If one is not available, use an ordinary table, or an old wooden door or worktop, and cover the surface with some form of padding. Alternatively, you can use a couch, a bed, a chair or the floor.

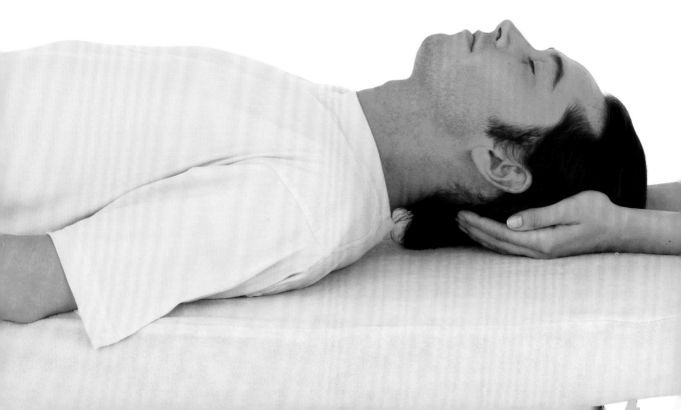

A SHORT PRAYER

Repeat (either silently or out loud) a short prayer or invocation. This is to remind yourself that you are a channel for this healing treatment and to express your gratitude. This enables you to recall that the healing energy is not coming from you and that it is not up to you. You can create your own prayer, or it can be something like this:

'We are asking the universal life force called Reiki to shower its light, love and healing energy on ... [name of receiver] for his/her highest and greatest good; and we are grateful for this.'

You can give Reiki treatment either sitting down or standing up – choose according to what feels the most comfortable for you personally.

TREATMENT GUIDELINES

- Create a safe, quiet environment (switch off the phone).
- Remove watches and jewellery (both giver and receiver).
- Remove shoes, belts and glasses, and loosen tight clothing (receiver only).
- Keep legs uncrossed (both receiver and giver).
- Use a pillow under the receiver's head and knees (if requested).
- Play soothing, meditative music, or treat in complete silence.
- Have a blanket and tissues nearby.
- Centre yourself (see page 58) either in the second (sacral) or fourth (heart) chakra.
- Ask about any disorders or surgery (see page 62).
- Explain briefly how Reiki works.
- Say a silent prayer to express your gratitude and remind yourself that you are a channel for Reiki energy (see page 59).
- Wash your hands before and after treatment.
- Smooth the aura (see page 62) before and after each treatment.
- Guide the receiver into a brief relaxation using the breath as a focal point
- Refrain from talking during treatment (see page 62).
- Stay in each position for three to five minutes.
- Do not remove your hands abruptly from the receiver's body.
- Let the receiver rest at the end of the treatment (see page 63).
- Offer a glass of still water after the treatment.
- Share what you noticed during the treatment (see page 63), without trying to make a diagnosis or suggesting medication; if appropriate, recommend that the receiver sees a doctor.
- Treat for a minimum of three to four consecutive daily treatments (see page 63) – continue with Reiki until the energy is balanced.

Treatment positions

Try sitting down while treating, and select a chair that is the right height for you; alternatively, treat while standing up – whatever feels best for you. However, be aware that kneeling or working hunched over will not be comfortable. Give the receiver pillows for the head and knees, especially if they have lower back problems. A cushion under the knees can help to release and relax any tension while lying on the back. When the person turns over to enable the back to be treated, place the cushion under the ankles.

Practicalities

Always keep a box of tissues, and a blanket or shawl nearby, so that you can cover the receiver if they get chilly. Wash your hands before and after treatment (in cold, running water after treatment to clear any negative energies). Take off your watch and any jewellery, so that

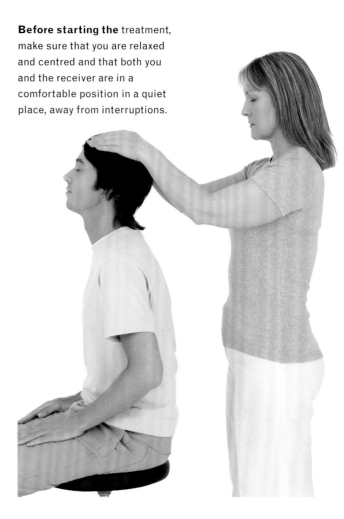

Before starting the treatment, make sure that you are relaxed and centred and that both you and the receiver are in a comfortable position in a quiet place, away from interruptions.

they do not disturb you during treatment, and ask the receiver to remove any shoes, glasses, jewellery and belts, and to loosen tight clothing – getting undressed is not necessary, because Reiki energy passes through all materials. Both giver and receiver should keep their legs uncrossed, so that the energy can flow freely.

Your hands

When placing your hands over the receiver's eyes, as in Head Position One (see page 134), spread a tissue over the eyes, if requested. Lay your hands on gently and lightly. Do not apply pressure to the receiver's body and keep your fingers together, since spread-out fingers scatter the energy. It is also important not to remove your hands abruptly when changing from one hand position to the next. Be aware that you are in intimate contact and the receiver is vulnerable; any sudden movement could cause a disturbance in their body and mind.

'Before I did the First Degree I kind of knew that I had to do something with my hands. But it always took an effort to do so. Now, having done the First Degree, this has changed utterly. There is no effort any more. Often I notice a feeling of warmth or a kind of tingling in my hands when giving Reiki to myself or to others. It feels really good. Reiki feels very "normal" to me now. I also realized that animals are easily affected by Reiki.'

Sam

Relax and centre yourself before starting treatment by placing your hands in the middle of your chest to connect with your heart centre (fourth chakra).

A complete Reiki treatment

For a complete Reiki treatment allow about an hour, depending on the receiver's ailments. As soon as your hands connect with the receiver's body, they sense the energy of that area and your hands 'know' how long they need to remain there (see pages 134–140 for the hand positions).

Asking for information

When treating someone for the first time, it is helpful to be aware of any disorders or surgery, to understand why the receiver is seeking Reiki or what their goal is. Sharing information is helpful to both of you. Ask in a general way, such as: 'Is there anything you would like me to know before we start?' Then listen and be open to what the receiver says, without trying to interpret or judge. Ask

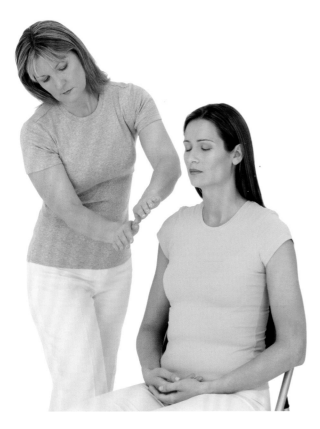

Smoothing the receiver's aura will have a calming effect and prepares him or her for the treatment. Afterwards, it helps to settle or dispel excess or negative energies.

only to gain more clarity, rather than to solve a problem. Mention possible self-healing reactions – a good sign, indicating that healing is taking place (see page 64).

Smoothing the aura

At the beginning and end of the treatment, smooth the receiver's aura three times, from above the top of the head down over and beyond the feet. Any disturbing energies in the aura can be released and the receiver will feel calmer. After treatment, hold both feet at the ankles for a moment, to ground the receiver. During the treatment Reiki will have activated and released energy from the physical body into the aura, and this might still be present. After the treatment, smoothing the aura helps the energies to settle and removes negative energy. The last stroke is upwards – from the feet over the top of the head – and helps the receiver to come back from the deep relaxation of the treatment more easily.

Guided relaxation at the outset

At the beginning of the treatment, guide the receiver into a brief relaxation using the breath as a focal point. Tell the receiver to imagine, with each out-breath, their body sinking deeper into the surface beneath them and breathing out mentally whatever they do not need at this moment (thoughts, worries, emotions, body tension).

Staying silent

It is important to carry out Reiki healing in silence. When giving or receiving Reiki we enter a deeper state of consciousness. We are open and connected to our intuition and may receive insights. Some people see vivid colours or bright lights, have images and memories (even of past lives) and get in touch with emotions or experience a spontaneous balancing in the body. Talking may be distracting and cause the receiver to miss the experience of this deeper level of consciousness (even though the Reiki energy is still taking effect).

Gassho meditation

Usui carried out this meditation with his students before treatment to strengthen the flow of Reiki energy. The Japanese word *Gassho* means 'two hands coming together'. The meditation can be used as a preparation for treatment and as a centring exercise. It focuses on the hands and the heart chakra, and is intended to bring the giver into a meditative state, providing the active mind with a structure and focus to enable it to calm down. You can do this meditation daily, morning or evening, for about 10–20 minutes or longer.

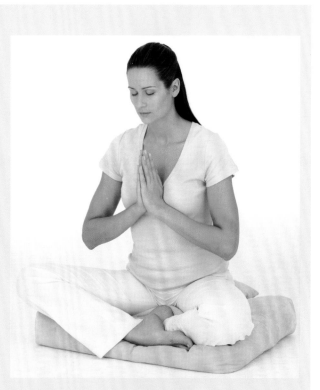

1 Sit with your eyes closed and back straight (lean against a wall or use a cushion). Allow your breath to flow in and out naturally, and relax.

2 Now fold your hands together and hold them comfortably in front of your chest. Breathe in through the nose and out through the mouth, so that the out-breath touches the fingertips like a breeze – perhaps adjust the height of your hands to make this possible.

3 Place your tongue on the roof of your mouth when you breathe in; on the out-breath, place your tongue at the bottom of your mouth.

4 Now pay full attention to the point where your two middle fingers meet – and forget everything else.

After the treatment

At the end of the treatment, let the receiver rest for about 5–10 minutes, then help them come back slowly to normal consciousness. Offer a glass of water to help the body release any toxins. Ask how the receiver feels and share whatever you became aware of during the treatment. Perhaps you noticed sensations in your hands, such as hot, cold or tingling, or the shifting of energy (see page 65). Pointing out what you have perceived is valuable, but do not diagnose or prescribe.

Problem areas

During a full Reiki treatment you can treat problem areas separately for about 10–20 minutes. You might experience these areas as different sensations, such as tingling or throbbing in your hands, or a change of temperature from heat or cold in the receiver's body, or in your hands, might guide you. Give Reiki here until you sense that the temperature and energy flow have normalized. Chronic complaints require intensive treatment over a prolonged period of time. With elderly or sick people, start with half an hour's treatment and then increase the time gradually. When treating babies or children, 10–20 minutes may be sufficient time.

A course of treatment

When you treat a receiver for the first time, ideally begin with three to four consecutive, daily Reiki treatments. This gives the body enough time to open itself on an energetic plane, so that it is able to free itself of toxins more effectively. As it does so, chronic disorders may again become acute. These are self-healing reactions and are part of the healing process. They usually subside within 2–24 hours (see page 64). The number and frequency of additional sessions can be determined after these initial treatments.

Healing responses and detoxification

Reiki healing begins with cleansing the body of toxins, stimulating the organs and nervous system, healing inflamed and contaminated areas of the body (bacteria and virus infections), loosening and removing blockages in the energy system and strengthening the generally available energy and immune system.

This back position – Back Position Three – is an effective detoxifier, and also strengthens the kidneys and adrenal glands as well as the nervous system.

Reactions

Each treatment works on different levels and produces a deep cleansing effect on the mind, body, emotions and spirit. Self-healing reactions are a part of the healing process and generally subside between two and 24 hours. They are a good sign and indicate that healing is taking place and that toxic energy is leaving the body. Drinking plenty of water or fluids (not coffee or black tea) is important to help the cleansing process.

First treatment

When someone receives Reiki for the first time it is advisable to give treatment daily, on four consecutive days or close together (perhaps two sessions in the same week). Reiki can stimulate healing reactions on the physical and emotional level. Usually after the first two sessions, detoxification of the physical body occurs. And after the third or fourth session, emotional blockages and feelings may be released and emotional responses may arise. It is helpful to let these feelings surface and be expressed. It is important to continue with Reiki and give further treatments once or twice a week, over a period of several weeks.

How long to hold each position

Energy tends to move in waves, pulsating. This can take a few minutes. Stay in each hand position until you feel that the receiver's body has absorbed all the energy it needs. Usually you will notice a feeling in your hands of having become 'normal' again and the energy will feel balanced. The giver may also experience reactions during the treatment. He or she is a channel for healing and is transmitting the Reiki energy. Allow these reactions to take place; energies can be transformed in this way.

RELEASING BLOCKS

Possible reactions in 'blocked' areas of the body:

- Yawning
- Coughing
- Hiccups
- Jerking
- Tingling in the hands
- Thirst

TREATMENT RESPONSES AND PERCEPTIONS

Possible healing responses for the receiver:

- Feeling chilly during or after the treatment, perhaps changing after ten minutes into a pleasant feeling of warmth
- An urgency to go to the bathroom (a positive sign of relaxation)
- Hunger and thirst
- Chronic ailments becoming more acute
- A feeling of pressure in the head, or a headache
- Emotional responses – usually after the third or fourth treatment
- Detoxification (showing in a change of consistency and colour of stools or urine)
- If a bone is broken, increased pain (showing that healing is starting)

Possible healing perceptions for the giver:

- Heat in the hands
- Tingling in the hands
- Vibration and shaking in the body
- A feeling of energy shifting beneath the hands
- A feeling of energy being drawn (or pulled) in
- Heat and perhaps sweating in the body
- Coldness beneath the hands (usually an indication of a chronic ailment)

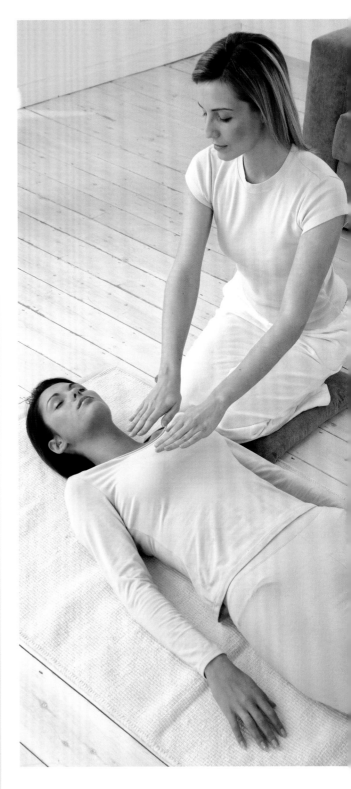

As the giver, you are the channel through which the healing energy is transmitted to the receiver, so you may also feel physical reactions to the treatment.

The attunement process

As we have seen, an attunement (also called 'energy-transmission') is the way in which Reiki is passed from Master to student. This happens during a sacred ceremony, which is a vital part of Reiki training.

The four attunements

In the First Degree, four separate attunements are given (over two days), in which the Reiki energy builds up slowly. The initiations into the First Degree mainly affect the physical body and the etheric energy body. This enables the receiver to absorb more Universal Life Energy and let it flow through the whole body.

The first attunement in the First Degree connects, on the physical level, the heart with the thymus gland. It also harmonizes the fourth chakra on the etheric level of the energy body. The second attunement takes effect on the thyroid gland. On the etheric body it supports the opening of the fifth chakra, the centre for communication.

The third attunement influences the pituitary gland and the hypothalamus, which is responsible for our moods and body temperature. On the etheric body it affects the sixth chakra.

The fourth attunement is connected to the pineal gland and affects the etheric level, the seventh chakra. This chakra is linked to Higher Intelligence (intuition) and opens the connection to the spiritual world. Each attunement triggers a form of cleansing, which is normal because the body and its energy system first need to adjust to the higher vibration of Reiki (see the 21-Day Cleansing Process, page 76).

'I regularly did daily self-treatment after the course and my mind gained clarity. It is easier for me to take decisions now and I can see my goals clearly. I have an enjoyable sense of well-being. If I cannot treat myself with Reiki, because of lack of time, I really feel that something is missing!'

Sabine

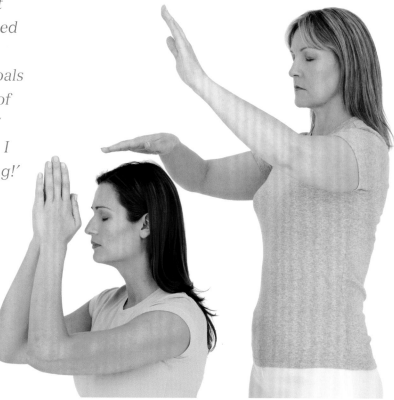

The student receives four separate 'energy-transmissions' in a gradual build-up of healing Reiki energy. These attunements increase the vibration frequency of the four upper chakras.

The effects of attunement

Being initiated into First Degree Reiki is a powerful spiritual experience, although the way it is experienced is different for each person. However, there are some common perceptions. For example, many students feel a stronger energy flow in the body, which often manifests itself as a pleasant wave-like flow and expansive feeling of warmth. Others see a bright light or a variety of vivid colours in their sixth (third-eye) chakra.

After attunement students experience a deeper emotional and spiritual encounter with themselves, and sometimes tears flow. Some people have personal insights or visions, and a space of peace, silence and meditation opens up. For many, the senses such as smell, hearing, sight and touch are enhanced. Whatever you experience (even if very little) is normal and, regardless of what you experience, your 'inner healing channel' is opened and you are attuned to the Reiki energy. Once you are attuned, you cannot lose this ability. Even after a break of several years you can immediately use the Reiki power again.

Previous experience

If someone has already done energy work (for example, martial arts, Qi Gong or Tai Chi) or other forms of healing, or if they meditate regularly, their energy bodies may already be attuned to higher energetic vibrations. They are able to absorb more Reiki energy and can channel more energy right from the start.

New to Reiki

For people to whom energy or spiritual work is new, they will still be able to channel Reiki (after attunement), but initially the sensations and the flow of energy they experience may be smaller. However, after a few weeks of practise (usually 6–8 weeks) they will experience the full flow of Reiki energy. At the beginning of your training it is important to practise as often as possible. The more you use the Reiki energy, the better it flows. After First Degree training it is recommended to give yourself at least three weeks of daily Reiki treatment.

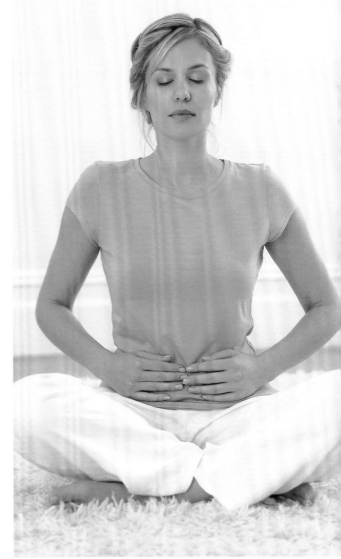

The first few weeks following the First Degree initiation is a key time in the consolidation of your Reiki training. Self-treatment should be maintained on a daily basis.

How to use the First Degree

First and foremost, use Reiki on yourself, daily, and then move on to help others. You will find all the Reiki hand positions for self-treatment in Chapter 6 (see pages 128–132). The more Reiki you give yourself, the better the healing energy is able to loosen up blockages and promote healing and deep relaxation on all levels. Through self-healing you become familiar with Reiki energy and any healing reactions.

Starting to treat others

You will intuitively know when it is time to start using Reiki on others. You will find all the Reiki hand positions for treating others in Chapter 6 (see pages 133–146). It is good to start with family members and friends, as Reiki offers a positive opportunity to spend time together in a secure atmosphere. Giving Reiki to your partner may enhance the quality of your relationship, too. Because you do not speak during Reiki, you enter another level of communication, without using the mind, which can deepen the way you relate to each other. The same is true for your relationships with children or parents: all feel the love and care they receive through you and through Reiki.

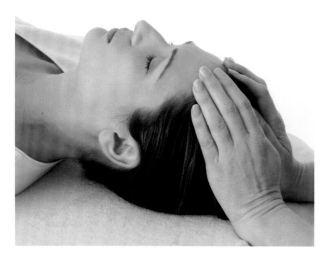

Move on to treating others when you instinctively feel that the time is right, and then begin with members of your family and friends, which can strengthen your relationships.

Short, informal treatments

You can give Reiki as a short treatment for half an hour on a chair (see pages 147–151). This is good if there is inadequate time for a full treatment and you want to ease a stressful situation, release tension or a headache, recharge or refresh energy and balance the energies of the chakras. Using Reiki with friends and colleagues can improve your relationships with them, too. Reiki opens the door for both giver and receiver to connect.

Group treatment

You can give Reiki in a group of three, four, six or even more people. You share the energy with other Reiki channels and the treatment time is usually shorter than for a normal treatment. The Reiki power flows more intensely and the effect lasts longer. In a group of Reiki friends, one person lies down and is treated by each of the others in turn (see pages 152–155).

Daily self-treatment

Make it part of your routine to give yourself Reiki at specific times of the day, for example in the mornings: an ideal way to begin each new day. You can do a full self-treatment or take 20–30 minutes to treat your head and front. If you do not have that much time, at least put your hands for ten minutes on whichever part you feel needs attention. Try treating the back of the head the moment you wake up (see opposite). This will help gently return you to normal waking consciousness, especially if you have problems waking and then getting up.

During the day, at odd moments such as when you are making a phone call, watching television or waiting for something, lay your hands on your body and intentionally use Reiki energy. If you have problems getting to sleep, an evening treatment can also be very beneficial.

Morning Reiki self-treatment

If you feel unsettled or moody, treating yourself with Reiki will immediately change your frame of mind, improving your outlook on the day. The following treatment will wake you up gently and prepare you.

Maintain each of the hand positions specified in turn for around 3–5 minutes, or for as long a time as you sense that the Reiki energy is being absorbed and feels beneficial for you.

Instructions

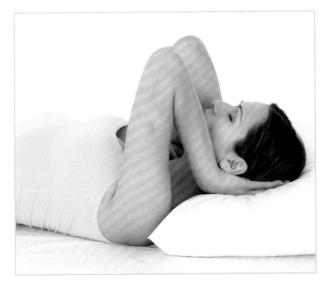

1 Lay your hands on the back of the head, holding your head like a ball, fingers pointing upwards, in Head Position Four.

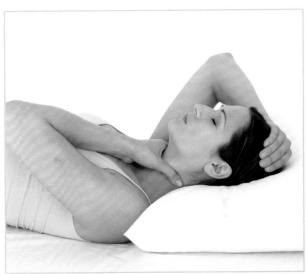

2 Place one hand on the centre of the top of the head, and lay the other directly on the front of the throat, over the thyroid gland.

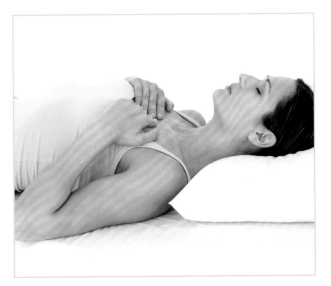

3 Continue treating your heart, placing your hands on either side of your upper chest, fingers touching, just below the collarbone, in Front Position One.

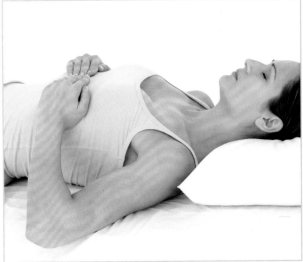

4 Place your hands over the lower ribcage, above the waist, fingers touching in the middle, using Front Position Two.

Reiki self-treatment before going to sleep

Reiki self-treatment has a calming effect on body, mind and soul, as well as harmonizing all your chakras. You can also use this treatment effectively any time you need a sense of calm and peace. It works best if you have difficulty getting to sleep or cannot get back to sleep.

Keep your hands in each position for 3–5 minutes. If you happen to fall asleep during the treatment, don't worry; you might want to finish it the following morning. You can do this treatment in silence or play gentle, relaxing music.

Instructions

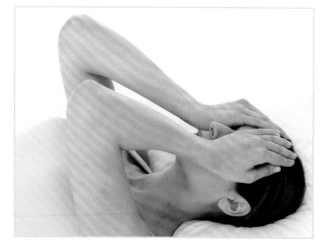

1 Place your hands over your eyes, resting your palms on your cheekbones, in Head Position One. This connects you with your intuition.

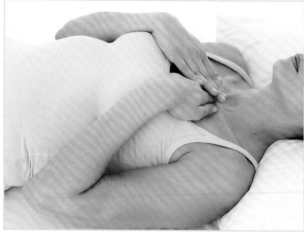

2 Place both hands on the middle of your chest – the seat of your heart chakra. This will strengthen your immune system and increase your capacity for love and the enjoyment of life.

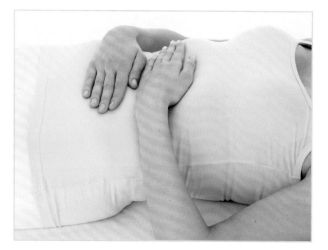

3 Place one hand on your solar plexus and the other just below it – touching your stomach – allowing yourself to relax deeply into this area, and letting healing energy flow throughout your whole body.

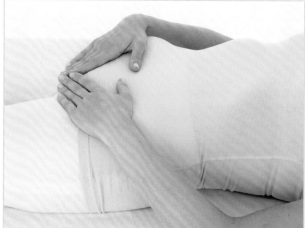

4 Place both hands in the shape of a V over your lower abdomen, with the fingertips touching over the pubic bone, in Front Position Four. This provides grounding and encourages you to trust more in life, which allows sleep to come more easily.

First Degree cleansing process

After taking the First Degree, cleansing and clearing usually take about three weeks (see also pages 50 and 76). This process happens after each Reiki degree.

Higher rate of vibration

The Reiki attunements amplify the vibratory frequency of the physical body and the subtle energy bodies of the aura. This can happen quite suddenly in specific areas – physically, emotionally, mentally and spiritually. Negative energies can arise and then need to be released. Energy blockages and hardened patterns vibrate more slowly than positive feelings, such as love and joy. The clearing process occurs through the chakras. Even though the opening of the Reiki channels is between the heart and the crown chakra, the lower chakras (first, second and third) are equally involved in this process of clearing, harmonizing and balancing. Usually each chakra takes about three days to adjust itself to the higher frequency of vibration. For the seven main chakras the whole process takes about 21 days.

First Degree cleansing reactions

During the cleansing process certain personal issues might reappear, perhaps through dreams, memories, thoughts, people or circumstances; or strange 'old' moods might resurface, or emotional changes, physical symptoms and toxins might be released. Reiki can bring up feelings, negative thoughts and sometimes physical imbalances, especially if an illness has been concealed beneath the surface. Whatever has been 'kept back' and is ready to be encountered, in order to be healed, can now surface. On the physical level temporary healing reactions might include headaches, a cold or profuse sweating, occasionally nausea, overnight fever or diarrhoea.

Accepting changes

Initially, these reactions may be uncomfortable, especially if we resist them. The best strategy is to welcome them as a 'healing crisis'. Accept each experience without clinging to it or worrying about it; it will disappear naturally, spontaneously, usually when you let go of it. It might be helpful to write things down in a journal. Perhaps record your dreams, memories, insights, feelings, inner changes and experiences during self-treatment, plus anything else you become aware of during the 21 days.

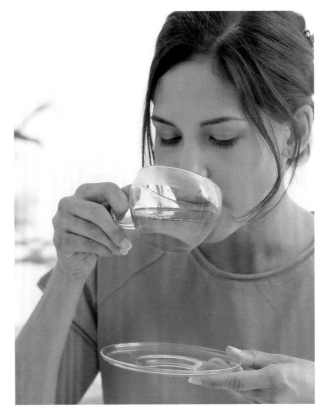

During the cleansing process, it is advisable to limit your intake of caffeine-containing black tea and coffee in favour of plenty of still water and herbal teas.

To support this cleansing process, daily self-treatment is very important, in order to advance and refine your own energy, enhancing your spiritual growth. Let go of any mental or emotional obsessions and allow a feeling of gratitude to enrich you. As always, drink plenty of still water or herbal teas during this period (at least 2–3 litres/3½–5 pints a day) and try to reduce, or avoid altogether, your intake of toxins such as alcohol, cigarettes and recreational drugs, and perhaps drink less tea and coffee.

Treating animals with Reiki

You can help your pet feel better and boost its immune system with Reiki. Most animals seem to love Reiki and respond very well to it. They feel something special emanating from your hands, becoming calm and relaxed as a result.

Where to treat

Usually animals show you, with their body position, where to place your hands. For example, your dog (or cat) might roll onto its back to urge you to place your hands on its belly. Pay attention to areas that draw more energy, as this can indicate an imbalance. If you own fish, place

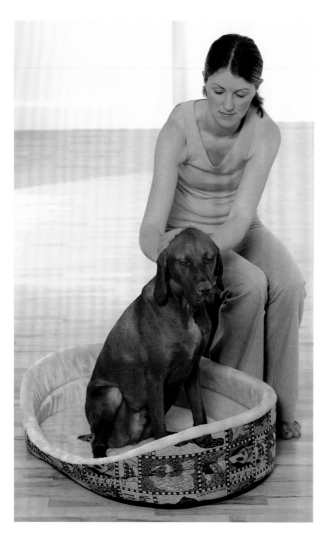

your hands around the tank or over the pond. For a small caged animal or bird, simply hold it in your hands or place your hands around the cage.

The position of organs in mammals is very similar to that of humans. Treat your pets (dogs and cats) and domestic animals (cows, horses) behind the ears. Horses are very receptive to Reiki, which usually calms their nerves. You can place one hand on top of the head and the other under the throat; this gives a feeling of comfort. Treat the chest, stomach, back and hips for ailments such as stomach upsets or arthritis. Treat painful spots or specific injuries directly, concentrating on that area. Treat over plaster in the case of a broken bone. Some hand positions will depend on where you are able to reach or where the animal allows you to touch. Remember: Reiki always flows to the area that most needs it.

Practical guidelines

Cats and dogs tend to remain lying down for as long as they need Reiki. They let you know when they have had enough by changing position or jumping away. Between ten and 30 minutes' treatment is usually enough. Reiki also helps to calm your pet while you are waiting to see the vet or during the examination.

For animals that have undergone an operation, a daily Reiki treatment can speed recovery. Before an operation or an anaesthetic, Reiki is helpful to calm the animal, and it also helps them recover far more quickly from the side-effects of anaesthetic afterwards.

For First Degree initiates, the following method is an alternative way to send Reiki at a distance. Stand a safe distance away, place your hands in the direction you want the healing energy to flow and send the Reiki intentionally. You can also send Reiki through your own aura into the auric energy field of the animal.

Most animals usually like being touched on the head – try behind the ears, under the chin and in the middle of the forehead above the eyes.

Using Reiki on plants, food and drink

Plants, seeds and flowers respond very well to Reiki energy, helping them to stay healthy, grow faster or recover from a specific problem. And because Reiki helps us to become more in touch with what our body really needs, you can also use it to enrich food and drink.

Techniques for treating plants

Potted plants can be treated by putting your hands around the entire pot (for a minute or two), just as if you were giving treatment to a person. You can also hold your hands 15 cm (6 in) away from the plant and send healing energy towards it. Treat the leaves by placing your hands around them. When you transplant any plant, growth can be affected as you move it. It is best to treat the plant before uprooting it and treat the roots before you put the plant into its new location. You can give Reiki to plants' water, too, by holding your hands over the watering can or when you are holding a hosepipe.

If you have a garden, you can treat seeds with Reiki before planting them. Hold them in your hands (or treat the whole packet) for one or two minutes, letting your hands carry Universal Life Energy to the seeds. After planting, return in the coming days and place your hands on the trays and soil covering the seeds. You can treat cut flowers by placing your hands around the stems or vase. Encourage herbs and vegetables to grow stronger and more quickly by placing your hands around them.

Enriching food and drink

You can enrich, cleanse and energize food and drink, simply by holding your hands over or around the items just before you eat or drink them. Keep your hands in place for 30–60 seconds, sending out Reiki energy intentionally. Adding Reiki not only enhances the nutritional value of your food, but can also balance the negative side-effects of additives, preservatives and other chemicals. When you are eating out, you can discreetly hold your hands either on the side of the plate or above it, or around your cup or glass. Keep your hands in position for 15–30 seconds, focusing your intention on Reiki flowing into the food and drink.

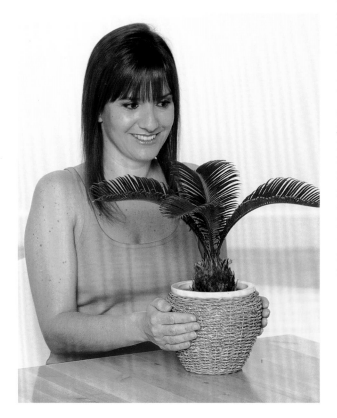

Give Reiki to the roots of potted plants by placing your hands around the pot. You can also treat an injured area, such as a stem, directly by putting your hands around it.

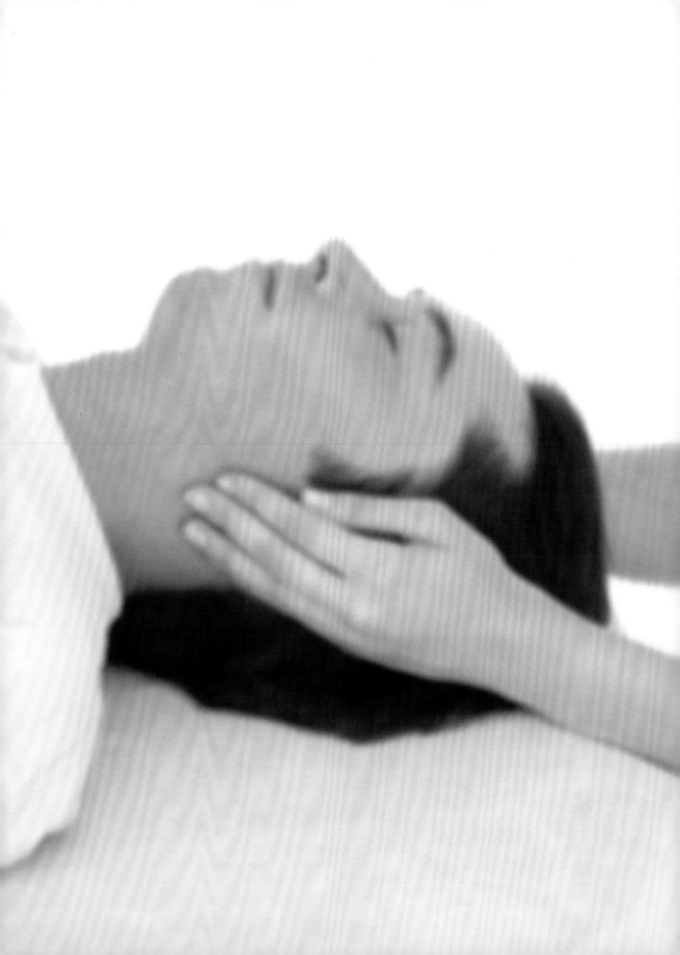

The Second Degree

The Second Degree broadens your Reiki knowledge and healing skills, and supports you in your inner growth and spiritual development. It is recommended for all those who want to explore their personal development further and experience the healing energies of Reiki on deeper levels. You will become attuned to and learn the Reiki symbols, their meaning and use in daily life and for specific healing situations. You will also be shown special healing methods, such as Mental Healing and Distant Healing.

Preparation for the Second Degree

Allow at least 2–3 months of practice between the First and Second Degree attunements. Take as much time as you feel you need, so that your body can adjust and get used to the higher vibrations set in action by the energy attunements of the First Degree.

You can take the Second Degree months, or even years, after the First. It is important to have plenty of Reiki experience after taking the First Degree. You also need to process what has happened to your body on both the physical and energetic planes. Regular self-healing and the desire to experience the Reiki energy on deeper levels are indicators as to when you are ready to go on to Second Degree training.

Why take the Second Degree?

If you wish to use Reiki healing professionally, it is strongly recommended that you take the Second Degree, as your Reiki energy becomes much stronger and you then become a wider channel for healing energy to flow through. In addition, it is well worth learning the Second Degree techniques for healing others on deeper levels in relation to emotional and mental problems.

How a Master-Teacher judges readiness

The Master-Teacher responsible for initiation into the Second Degree has to find the student 'trustworthy' enough to receive the Reiki symbols and the empowerment they give. He or she has to evaluate the student as being 'ready' for this next step, and being willing to respect and honour the tradition of Reiki and the sacredness of the symbols. The student needs to realize the value of the symbols and the responsibility carried by using them for the highest good of all.

How to select a Master-Teacher

From the student's viewpoint, the Master-Teacher should be someone he or she feels drawn to and who can be trusted. This involves personal intuition, but checks should also be made as to what Reiki training and lineage the Master-Teacher has and the content of their Second Degree training. After Mrs Takata's death, various branches and dilutions of Usui Reiki appeared (see page 17). This brought differences in interpretation and some

21-DAY CLEANSING PROCESS FOR THE SECOND DEGREE

The cleansing and clearing process takes place after each Reiki degree and lasts about three weeks. The Second Degree attunement is very powerful because you receive empowerment with the three Reiki symbols. It affects the physical body as well all the energy centres (chakras) of the energy body. The first chakra, in particular, receives strong stimulation and helps to clear any issue you might have with survival and sexuality. It can also stimulate a physical healing reaction, such as a short-lived overnight fever or a feeling of the onset of flu, which soon dissipates. The attunement stimulates your sixth chakra and strengthens intuition, supporting spiritual growth.

To support this 21-day cleansing process, daily self-treatment is very important and will advance and refine your energies. Drink plenty of still water or herbal teas (around 2–3 litres/3½–5 pints a day) and try to reduce your intake of alcohol, tobacco, drugs and caffeine.

misunderstandings of Reiki teaching. The right symbols and their dynamic use are important for effective results with the methods taught in the Second Degree. True Reiki includes the inner growth of consciousness and spiritual development as part of healing.

Preparation

If self-treatment is not yet part of your routine, two weeks prior to the training, start giving yourself daily Reiki treatment to open you up to receiving the tools, teachings and energy-transmissions of the Second Degree.

The Master-Teacher needs to assess that a student is ready to move on to the Second Degree. For their part, the student should feel that the Master-Teacher is 'right' for them.

What you learn in the Second Degree

The Second Degree training introduces further aspects of the inner exploration of the self and spiritual development, using a variety of methods. It is usually taught over a weekend, or two days, but it can also be taught over four consecutive evenings. Traditionally, the Second Degree was taught over four sessions, each lasting about three hours.

Training attunements

On the first morning you receive the Second Degree initiation. This comprises a single attunement. This energy-transmission sets a great deal in motion on all levels (mental, physical, emotional and spiritual) and is much more powerful than the First Degree attunements because the vibratory rate is about four times stronger. The transmission allows more Reiki energy to flow through you and has a particular effect on the etheric body (the second energy body) and the chakras. The pituitary gland (the sixth chakra) is stimulated, which greatly enhances your intuition and healing ability. The Second Degree attunement empowers you to work with the three sacred Reiki symbols (comprising a pictorial representation and a name or 'mantra', see opposite), which are the main tools for the Mental Healing and Distant Healing techniques.

The Mental Healing technique is used for dealing with deep-seated emotional and mental problems. The Distant Healing method is a highly effective absentee healing technique and can be used to send remotely. The healing energy is sent on a mental level to any living thing – whether human, animal or plant – or to any problem or difficult situation that requires healing. You also receive the knowledge and usage of the three Reiki symbols and their mantras (sacred Sanskrit words and sounds that set subtle energies in vibration).

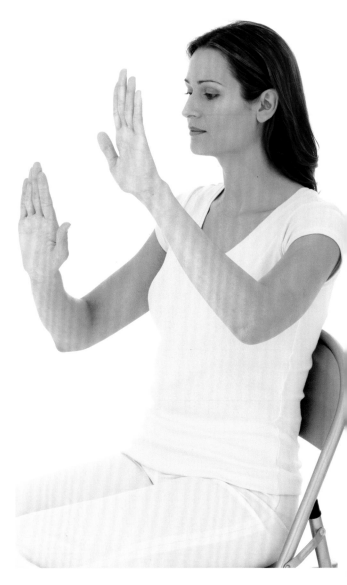

Second Degree training enhances your healing ability, enabling you to work with the Reiki symbols in using the Distant Healing technique.

The Reiki symbols and mantras

The Usui method of Reiki employs four symbols in total: three are given during the Second Degree and the fourth symbol is given during the Third Degree. These symbols are expressed as calligraphic drawings and are always used in conjunction with their corresponding mantras.

Origins

The origin of these symbols goes back to the ancient Buddhist scriptures, where Usui found the symbols written in Sanskrit (see page 14). The third symbol comprises Japanese Kanji (the Japanese system of writing). All the symbols – which can be hand-drawn or visualized to any size, large or small – possess a three-dimensional form and carry metaphysical energy. When they are drawn they vibrate at a great rate.

Activation of the symbols

The first three Reiki symbols (the Power, Harmony and Distance Symbols) are only revealed and taught to students of the Second Degree. The fourth Reiki symbol (the Master Symbol) is part of the Third (or Master) Degree (see pages 116–119). Each symbol is activated through empowerment of the attunement process. Reiki energy can flow perfectly well without the symbols (as in the First Degree), but use of the symbols adds power to Reiki healing and makes its energy much stronger. Depending on which symbols are used, the energy is directed towards different healing approaches, such as Mental and Distant Healing. Each symbol is easy to use and works automatically when applied and activated.

Confidentiality

The Reiki symbols are sacred and transferred personally from Master to student. Unless someone has been officially attuned and empowered with each symbol, they cannot activate Reiki and its higher power. It is part of the Reiki tradition that the symbols are kept confidential, since they are powerful tools. They embody and activate divine forces and are therefore not transferred lightly or thoughtlessly. Some Masters have published the symbols in books or on the Internet. Apart from breaching confidentiality, these sources have been found to contain errors. In this book the Reiki tradition of confidentiality is honoured and the symbols are not printed.

When you are learning the symbols in a Second Degree training session, you usually draw them on paper, for practice. But as soon you are familiar with them, you trace them in the air in front of you. The idea is that the symbols are vibrant and transcendental, rather than stagnant on paper. You can also visualize them from your inner eye – your third eye (sixth chakra) – or trace them inside your mouth with your tongue.

Function and uses of the symbols

The Reiki symbols are like keys that open doors to higher levels of consciousness: beyond time and space. They increase the student's awareness and develop their intuition, sensitivity and ability – for example, to pick up messages in the receiver's subtle energy bodies. In this way, problems and imbalances on a physical, mental, emotional or spiritual level can be detected far more quickly and easily. With the tools learnt in the Second Degree, Reiki can work on deeper levels, to discover the real reason underlying illness or imbalance.

The Power Symbol (also known as the First Symbol) can be widely used in daily life and can also be easily integrated, greatly enhancing the healing energy of a normal Reiki treatment. The Harmony Symbol (also known as the Second Symbol) helps deal with deep-seated emotional and mental problems. And the Distance Symbol (also called the Third Symbol) sends the healing energy on a mental level, beyond space and time, to another person at a distance. Distant Healing can also be used to send healing and positive, loving thoughts to any difficulty in life: either in the past (which can now be healed) or to a future situation (which can be positively energized and influenced).

Each Reiki symbol has a corresponding, confidential mantra. The Power and Harmony Symbols both have a three-syllable mantra and the Distance Symbol has a five-syllable mantra. Each mantra is repeated three times after the symbol has been drawn or visualized in golden light.

The Power Symbol and its application

The Power Symbol is the first symbol, enhancing the power of Reiki and bringing the energy into the present moment. In translation the symbol mantra means 'All the energy of the universe: be present'. This brings the energy of the universe to the earth.

Function

The main function of this symbol is to increase available energy. The Power Symbol can either be used alone or in combination with the Harmony and Distance Symbols in order to strengthen them. In the latter case, it is usually drawn behind the other two symbols, to activate the power of Reiki and make the vibration of each symbol stronger. Its main functions are to strengthen the healing energy, both cleansing and protecting it. Whenever it is used, this symbol of Reiki energy is transmitted. It can, for example, be visualized directly onto a person as a kind of blessing.

'All the energy of the universe: be present.'

Uses of the Power Symbol

You can use the Power Symbol to centre yourself – for example, before giving a treatment. Trace the symbol in front of you in the air, additionally visualizing it in golden light, and say the mantra three times. Keep your hands up and hold the energy for 1–2 minutes, feeling the effect that the symbol has on you.

Cleansing a treatment room

You can cleanse your treatment room using the Power Symbol. Trace the symbol in front of you in the air, let the Reiki energy flow out of both palms into the room and direct your hands towards the area you want to be cleared of negative energies. You can carry out this cleansing process in each corner of the room, the ceiling and the floor. Each time, repeat the sacred mantra three times. In addition, you can visualize a beam of white light emanating from both palms.

Changing the energy

The Power Symbol changes the energy of a place or of an item in a positive way. This is particularly important if you are staying away from home, perhaps in a hotel. You might also want to cleanse the energy of the bed by tracing the symbol onto it, visualizing it in golden light and saying the mantra three times. Keep your hands raised for 1–2 minutes. If you are working in a busy place, with many people and different energies, and want to keep the energy positive, visualize a huge Power Symbol spreading from the ceiling down to the floor and rotating. Keep the intention of Reiki and visualize the symbol moving in all directions, radiating light-energy onto everything. When you are cleansing an item, such as a crystal, healing stone or food, keep your hands around the item and let Reiki flow into it. In the case of food, this will also energize it positively, making it more digestible.

Protection

You can use the Power Symbol for personal protection. If you notice that the energy is negative in a crowd, do not trace the symbol in public, but simply visualize it in front of you, behind you, on each side, above and below you, as if you are in a box. If you want to protect someone else, visualize the symbol around that person, projecting the intention of protection and well-being.

This symbol is very helpful when travelling. In a car, trace or visualize the Power Symbol around it, in front, behind, on either side, above and below. On a long journey, visualize a big Power Symbol when you set out and let it move, in spirit, with you as you travel along. You can visualize the symbol in a train, bus or plane right up to your arrival. You can also trace the symbol along your route on a map and transmit the intention of experiencing a safe and enjoyable journey.

You can centre yourself and cleanse a room of any negative energies by tracing the Power Symbol in front of you and keeping your hands raised to allow the Reiki energy to flow out of your palms.

Reiki treatment using the Power Symbol

You can use the Power Symbol during your hands-on treatment to clear energies and to add Reiki energy to your treatment. The application of the symbol enhances the Reiki flowing through your hands as you place them on the receiver's body.

Starting off

When starting your treatment, trace the Power Symbol over the receiver's upper body before taking up a hand position. While you are giving treatment, you can trace the symbol over each new hand position before laying your hands on the specific area. This will clear any negative energy, loosen blockages and enhance Reiki power. It may be very beneficial to draw the Power Symbol over the top of the head (seventh chakra) and let Reiki flow into the receiver's aura, before starting the first hand position (covering the eyes).

Self-treatment

In Reiki self-treatment (when tracing the symbol on your own body), use the symbol in mirror image. When using the symbol on your front, start on the right side of your body. In this way, you will be sure to continue tracing in the correct direction. It is important that you do not reverse the symbol, as this will affect and change its whole purpose.

Enhancing awareness

Another quality of the Power Symbol is to enhance your own awareness. This is particularly beneficial when combining its use with either one or both of the other two Reiki symbols (see page 105). Here we put the Power Symbol between two or more people to increase awareness. This is also helpful when talking to another person and wanting to communicate from a higher level of consciousness.

Use the Power Symbol (First Symbol) over the receiver's body at the beginning of a Reiki treatment to centre the energy and give Reiki to the whole body.

The Harmony Symbol and its application

The Harmony Symbol is the Second Symbol and transmits qualities of harmony, peace and balance to the receiver. It especially affects the etheric body (second energy body) and its chakras. The translation of the symbol's mantra means 'Man and God are one'.

Mental and emotional uses

You can use the Harmony Symbol for mental and emotional problems going back to childhood. It is especially used for Mental Healing, to restore psychological and emotional balance and bring about peace and harmony. Through Mental Healing we make a connection between the three layers of the mind: the conscious mind (meaning 'man'), the unconscious or subconscious mind (meaning 'lower') and the superconscious mind, also known as the Higher Self (meaning 'higher') (see page 85).

The Harmony Symbol is used in the Mental Healing technique (see pages 87–89), drawn over the back of the receiver's head to connect the three layers of the mind (see page 85).

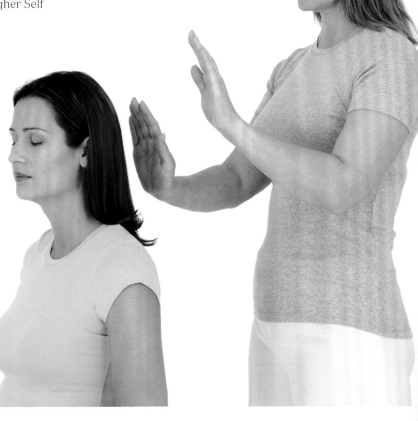

Physical uses

You can also apply the Harmony Symbol to the physical body, for example to areas that are overstimulated. The vibration of the symbol is absorbed by the etheric body and loosens blocked energy, balances and calms nervousness. This is particularly useful for the solar-plexus area (third chakra) and the chest area (heart/fourth chakra), relaxing and calming any emotional and disturbed energy. If there is a serious imbalance in the flow of energy, it is helpful to apply the symbol and give Reiki for at least three consecutive days. You can also use the Harmony Symbol to harmonize the quality of energy in a room. For example, after a social event you can apply the Harmony Symbol to balance and calm rotating energy.

Harmonizing the chakras

This is a gentle way to bring balance to another person's chakras or your own (when using self-treatment). Ask the receiver to lie comfortably on their back, eyes closed. Stay in each position long enough to sense the same amount of energy in both hands; this usually takes two or three minutes. You may feel tingling or pulsing sensations, too.

Instructions

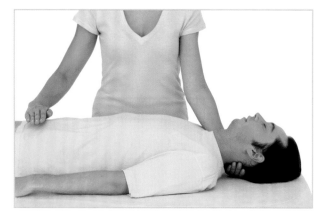

1 Lay one hand on the back of the receiver's head (this area is connected to the sixth chakra) and the other over the pubic bone (first chakra).

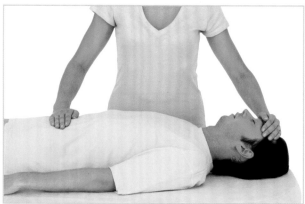

2 Place one hand on the forehead (sixth chakra) and the other below the navel (second chakra).

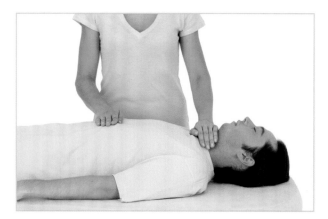

3 Lay one hand on the throat (fifth chakra) and the other on the solar plexus (third chakra).

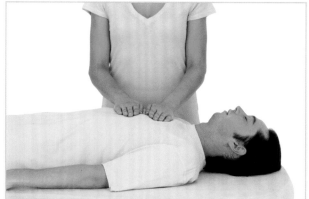

4 Now place both hands on the heart centre in the middle of the chest (fourth chakra), and allow Reiki to flow into the whole chest area.

The three layers of the human mind

It is known, from hypnosis and other metaphysical techniques and approaches, that the human mind consists of three main layers: the conscious mind, the unconscious mind and the superconscious mind.

The conscious and unconscious minds

The layer of the conscious mind (also called the ego) represents how we are normally identified by others and who we think we are. This layer is formed and influenced by parents, teachers, spiritual and religious experiences and by society itself. The conscious mind is formed from our thinking, speaking and behaviour, and from all our beliefs, attitudes, likes and dislikes – our whole personality. As we grow up, the conscious mind quickly learns what is right and what is wrong. It represses certain memories into the unconscious part of our mind, the subconscious. All that we feel to be 'wrong' has to be thrown into the 'basement' of the unconscious mind. Once things have been repressed, the unconscious mind gradually forgets about them. But it cannot directly release any of this repressed memory, such as fears, strong emotions (especially anger), belief systems or conditioning, because it is closed off, and the only way this can be achieved is to bring these memories back into the conscious mind.

The superconscious mind

If we go a little higher than the conscious mind we reach the superconscious layer. We may also call this our Higher Self, intuition, inner guidance, soul or spirit. It is alert and full of light. It knows clearly what our life purpose is and what is right for us. It is fully connected to the God/Goddess Consciousness and represents that wise part in us which provides us with deep insights and intuition. The superconscious loves and cares for us and for our highest good.

Mental Healing and the three layers

In Mental Healing, the three layers of the mind are connected. The superconscious mind can relieve the conscious mind of its conditioning and beliefs, and can allow the unconscious to release repressed memories through the conscious mind, by becoming aware of what is hidden beneath emotions, beliefs, fears and conditioning. The subconscious works with the superconscious. Together they direct messages and insights – for example, about the cause of an illness or other problems – to the conscious mind of the giver or receiver.

The Harmony Symbol is used to make contact with these hidden regions of consciousness and to work with deep-seated emotional problems, even going back through the years into childhood.

If you are told as a child that you are 'not good enough', 'stupid', 'good for nothing' or 'not lovable', after a period of time you will come to believe this and form a negative 'belief sentence' in your unconscious mind. In adult life, you might not consciously remember this 'belief sentence', but it still has a grip on you.

In Mental Healing you can consciously connect with your natural inner resources by applying healing affirmations. These describe a positive state that you wish for yourself. It can be just the opposite of your negative belief, such as 'I am good', 'I am intelligent' or 'I am lovable'. These inner resources strengthen your love for yourself, which can in turn help to resolve deep-seated emotional conflicts.

The following affirmation, or one like it, can be very powerful:

'I [name] love and accept myself, simply because I am as I am.'

This opens up your heart, and the burden of fighting and rejecting yourself may dissolve in a gentle, tearful manner. Speaking this affirmation brings you back closer to yourself, and you can then love and accept yourself again. This affirmation embraces all three areas of your being: mind, body and spirit.

Mental Healing

Mental Healing offers an opportunity to gain greater awareness about our past conditioning and programming, and encourages us to seek more clarity in life.

Uses of Mental Healing

Mental Healing can be used for fears, strong emotions, depression, sleeplessness, addictions like smoking or drugs, habits such as excessive eating or drinking, childhood issues and belief systems that we mostly carry unconsciously. Mental disturbances and negative beliefs about ourselves – such as 'I am not good enough', 'I can't do it', 'I am stupid' – prevent us from feeling good about ourselves and living life to its fullest potential. By giving Mental Healing, we can promote healing in the physical body and sometimes prevent a disease from appearing. When you want to know the cause of a disease, you can ask what the reason for it is and what the experience underlying this illness is. You can find out what you need to do to become fully healthy again.

Bringing light

Using the Mental Healing technique is like bringing light onto an issue or problem. For instance, you can use it if you have an unresolved mental or emotional problem or life pattern. You can ask the subconscious and superconscious minds to bring greater clarity and understanding into the conscious mind and request the programme, belief system or experience beneath to be revealed to you. You can also talk directly to the subconscious and find out whether there is a message for the conscious mind, and what someone needs to do to love, accept and heal themselves. The subconscious works with the superconscious and provides intuition, insights and clarity through dreams, pictures, visualizations, messages by means of words, instinctive 'gut' feelings, memories and so-called coincidences.

Giving Mental Healing

When giving Mental Healing to another person, you need to ask for their permission before you start. Never give Mental Healing without having asked the receiver first. This is important because you are in direct contact with all the various layers of the mind and divine intelligence: all becoming one. Therefore, you need to be a pure channel and try to keep your mind as empty as possible.

Usually, Mental Healing is given with the receiver sitting on a chair, with both feet on the ground next to each other. First, discuss the content (for example, whether the receiver wants guidance from their Higher Self); become clear what the issue or problem is, and what the person wants the healing for. Formulate a 'healing sentence', question or affirmation (a phrase or word describing a positive condition that the receiver desires) with the receiver, with the intention of healing. Repeat this silently and send it on a mental level inside the body of the receiver. In this way, the subconscious and superconscious become aware of the theme for the healing.

Next, tell the receiver that they might receive images, insights, feelings, accidental thoughts, impressions or answers, which might not make sense at first. They should just notice them and let whatever wants to happen occur. Messages and images can also be received in the giver's conscious mind. That is why it is important to discuss them afterwards. While the healing is in progress, trust and intend that this Reiki energy is channelled with love and light for the highest good of all involved.

'I enjoyed the attunement, and the atmosphere and the direct practice we did. The Mental Healing was very clearing and supportive. It helped me to accept and integrate an old, repressed part of me. I feel enriched somehow, more complete, and feel the desire to share and give.'

Frank

Instructions

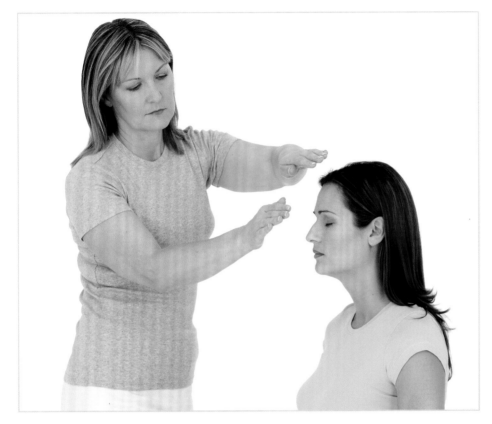

1 Smooth the aura of the receiver from above the head and shoulders down over the body.

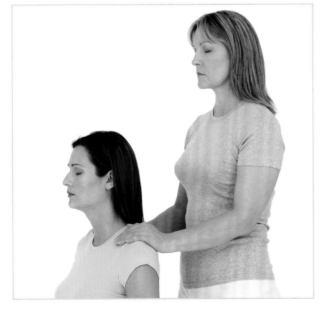

2 Draw a big Power Symbol over the back of the receiver. This stimulates Reiki energy and centres you. Then place both hands on top of the shoulders, for 30 seconds or so, to make a first connection with the receiver.

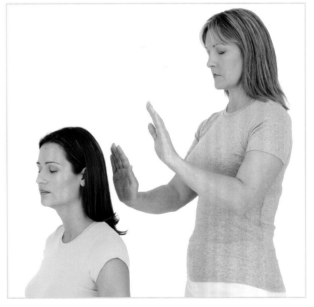

3 Now draw the Harmony Symbol on the back of the receiver's head, and behind you draw the Power Symbol, to give greater power.

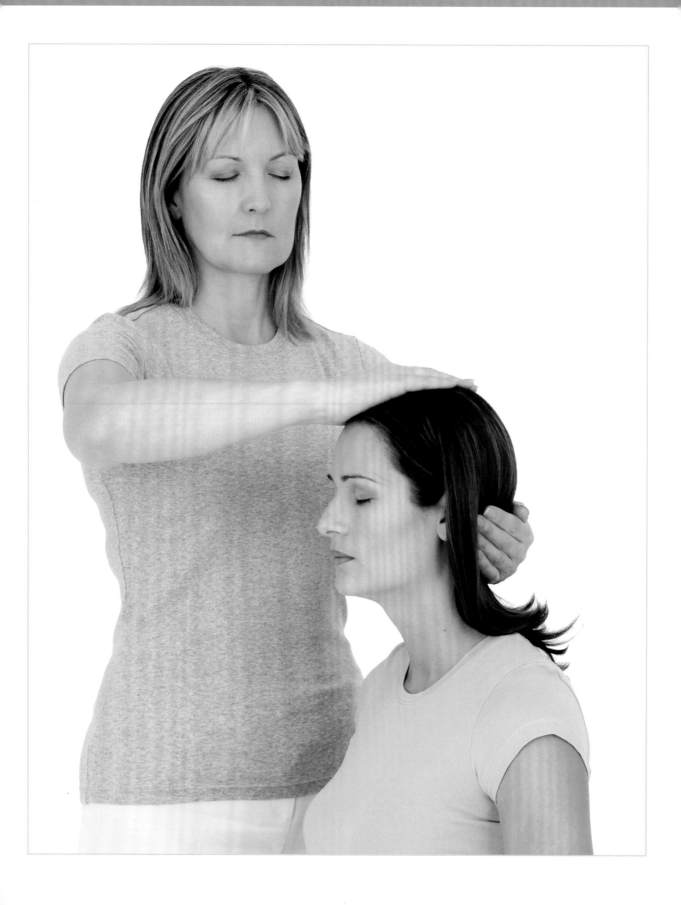

4 Place your dominant hand (usually the right hand) on top of the crown chakra and lay the other hand (usually the left hand) on the back of the head, with your palm covering the area where the head joins the neck. Keep your hands in these positions for the duration of the healing.

5 Now activate the symbols by visualizing them in golden light (first the Harmony Symbol, then the Power Symbol) and repeat their mantras three times. This opens up the link to the receiver's subconscious, conscious and superconscious layers, and establishes the connection between giver and receiver.

6 Now repeat the receiver's names three times silently (all names, including spiritual and childhood nicknames).

7 Fill yourself with light, love and energy by visualizing a beam of light entering the top of the head (crown chakra), flowing down through the throat, chest, torso and the whole body, down to the feet. Do this while you are breathing in.

8 On the out-breath, fill the receiver with light, love and energy by visualizing light, love and energy entering the top of your head first, then flowing into your arms and out through your hands into the receiver's body via the top of their head (crown chakra).

9 Establish a breathing rhythm, so that whenever you breathe in, you fill yourself with light, love and energy, and when you breathe out, you fill the receiver with light, love and energy. Do this for 2–4 minutes.

10 You might come across some areas that feel blocked, tense or are like dark 'corners' in the body. Send some extra light into those areas and notice where they are.

11 Now take your full attention to your inner eye (third-eye or sixth chakra) and keep your mind as empty as possible. If personal, accidental thoughts appear, ignore them and apologize for them. You can also imagine each thought passing by, like a cloud.

12 Now formulate your 'healing sentence', question or affirmation. Address the receiver's subconscious and superconscious directly.

13 Silently say: 'We ask the superconscious and subconscious of … [repeat the receiver's name] to make them aware of the reason for their problem … [name the problem] and show them what they need to do to love,

EXAMPLES OF HEALING SENTENCES

These are examples of healing sentences to connect to the superconscious and subconscious minds. Use them as they are, or change them according to the receiver's needs:

'We are asking the superconscious and subconscious of … [repeat the receiver's name]:

- To make them aware of the reason for their problem.
- To show them what they need to do to love, accept and heal themselves completely.

Keep the wording positive, because the subconscious cannot interpret negative words and phrases, such as 'not' and 'no'. You can also ask questions, such as: 'What is the experience and belief system beneath this issue or problem? Show me the next step I need to take in life.'

accept and heal themselves completely.' Repeat this sentence three times.

14 Then say out loud, 'The channel is open now', and wait. Maintain the hand position until you feel the process is complete. This usually takes 5–15 minutes.

15 At the end of the healing, send light, love, energy and thanks for receiving the healing, and find a way to mentally say 'goodbye'.

16 Finish the healing by gently parting your hands and rubbing them together to break the connection. Smooth the aura and make one stroke along the meridian on the back, down the spine, to refresh the energy.

Mental Healing during a Reiki treatment

Mental Healing can also be given to someone during a complete hands-on Reiki treatment.

Instructions

1 Start as you would for a normal Reiki treatment by laying your hands over the receiver's eyes, in Head Position One (see page 128).

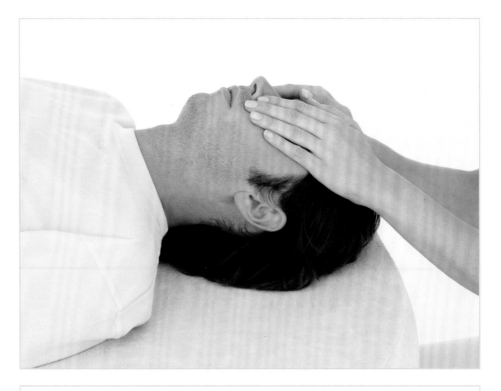

2 Again as in a normal Reiki treatment, place your hands either side of the head, above the ears, as in Head Position Two (see page 129).

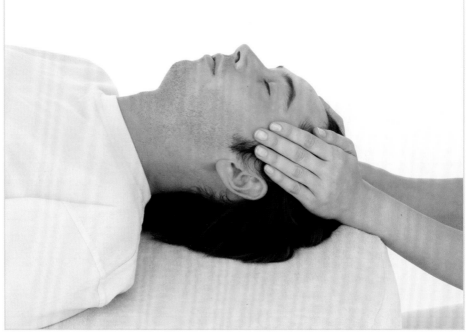

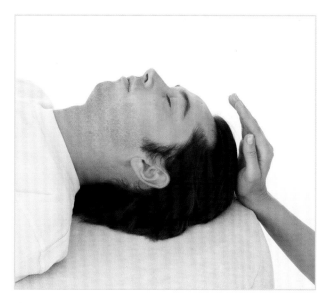

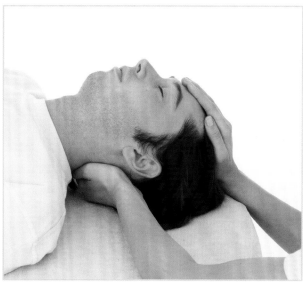

3 Apply the Mental Healing symbols. 'Draw' the Harmony Symbol behind the Power Symbol, over the top of the head (crown or seventh chakra).

4 Place the non-dominant hand (usually the left one) beneath the nape of the receiver's neck, with the palm touching the base of the skull, and the other hand (usually the right one) on top of the crown or seventh chakra. Visualize the symbols in golden light and say their mantras three times and the receiver's names three times. Continue with the Mental Healing steps already described (see page 89), from Step 8 – also sending light and love into the receiver's whole body – up to Step 16. This will take 5–10 minutes.

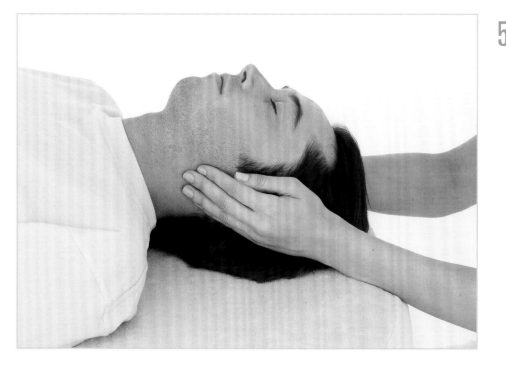

5 Remove your hands and continue with your normal Reiki treatment, either placing your hands on either side of the head, covering the ears, in Head Position Three (see page 129), or on the back of the head, holding the head like a ball, in Head Position Four (see page 129). Alternatively, you could move directly to treat the front.

Self Mental Healing

Mental healing is a powerful healing instrument and you can use it daily on yourself to deepen your connection with your own subconscious and superconscious (Higher Self).

Timing

A good time to do Mental Healing on yourself is in the morning when you have just woken up (and are still lying down) or at night before going to sleep. You can ask your Higher Self for guidance in bringing healing via the spirit. Allow about 10–15 minutes for the whole process.

You can also use this technique just to fill yourself with light, love and energy. This is a good way to gather and centre yourself at the end of the day. It gives you a pleasant feeling and keeps all the cells of your body vibrant. Try it for 5 minutes.

'Make me aware of the cause of my problem and show me what I need to do to love, accept and heal myself completely.'

Instructions

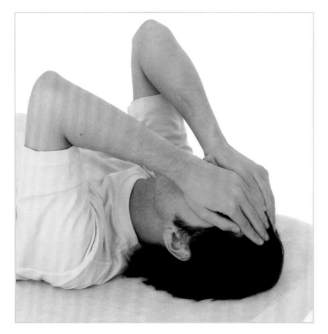

1 Lie or sit comfortably and relax. Cover your eyes with both palms and give Reiki for a few moments.

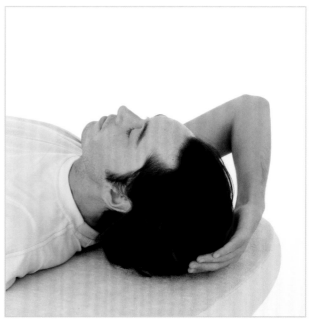

2 Now 'draw' the symbols over the back of your head (first the Harmony Symbol, then the Power Symbol).

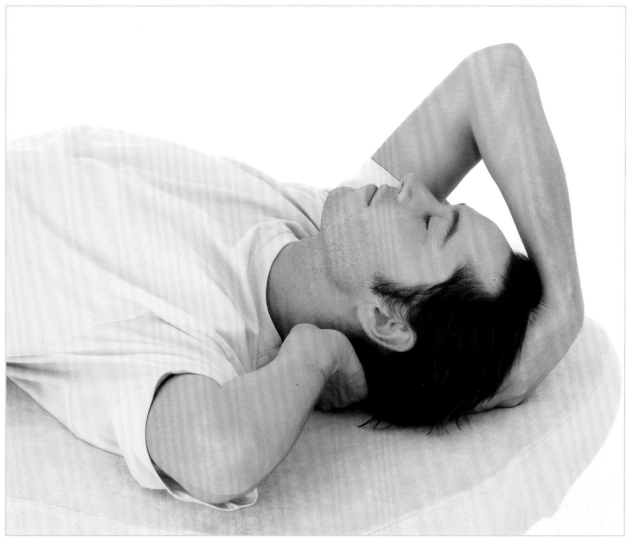

3 Place your right hand over your seventh chakra (on top of your head), with your fingertips pointing backwards, and place your left hand on the back of your head, with your palm covering the spot where your head joins your neck. Keep your hands here for the full length of the treatment.

4 Now activate the symbols and visualize them in golden light, seeing them entering your body through the top of your head (crown or seventh chakra). Repeat their corresponding mantras and your own full name three times.

5 Visualize a beam of light entering your body through your hands for a few minutes. Fill your whole body, from head to toe, with light, love and energy. Relax and enjoy the experience, feeling the wonderfully calming effect of the Harmony Symbol.

6 Now recall your 'healing sentence' or wish for guidance. Say silently inside, 'Make me aware of the cause of my problem … [mention the problem] and show me what I need to do to love, accept and heal myself completely.'

7 Repeat this three times and imagine the sentence entering your body through the top of your head.

8 Say out loud, 'The channel is open now, and waiting to receive further messages from the Higher Self.'

9 Become aware of any sensations in your body, or of any memories, images or feelings from your unconscious mind.

10 Before ending your healing, once again send light and love into your body, remove your hands gently and rub them together to break the connection.

The Distance Symbol and its application

The Distance Symbol is the Third Symbol and creates a connection with anything or anyone at a distance. The symbol comprises Japanese Kanji (the Japanese writing system) and consists of 22 strokes. In translation, the symbol means 'The God (Buddha/Christ) in me reaches out to the God (Buddha/Christ) in you, and we are one'. This means, in essence, that we form a connection between our own Higher Self and the Higher Self of others.

Function

The essence of the symbol is to send loving, healing energy on a mental level to a person, animal or plant, enabling you to connect with anything, anywhere, at any time. The Distance Symbol connects us to the sixth chakra and opens up intuition and strengthens the ability to 'see'. Communication from giver to receiver happens on this high level of consciousness, which is in touch with the Higher Self of both giver and receiver.

Uses of the Distance Symbol

This highly effective absentee healing technique will help you use energy in non-physical dimensions. You learn to send healing energy across a distance, beyond time and space. This is a transmission of light, transferring healing energy over a bridge of light to a distant recipient. It works similarly to radio-wave signal transmissions. The Distance Symbol makes the connection and 'fine-tunes' both sender and receiver for the healing.

This technique is very useful if you want to transfer vital healing to a friend or family member living away from you, or if you are travelling and want to send loving and healing energy to your pet at home. With Distant Healing you can send healing into the future or into the past. This is of great use when treating yourself or others, especially if, for example, a receiver is undergoing surgery and you want the healing to be received at a certain time in the future (after surgery). You can also send healing thoughts to any point in the past – to a difficult phase in childhood or an emotional and mentally upsetting event in your (or your receiver's) past (see page 105).

Other Distant Healing uses

With Distant Healing you can also send healing energy, light and loving thoughts to ongoing issues, such as the world's disasters and war zones. You can even send thoughts of peace and healing to flow to the whole planet. You can also use it to send relaxation, love and light to a dying person, especially if you cannot be present, as a way of saying goodbye to the departing person.

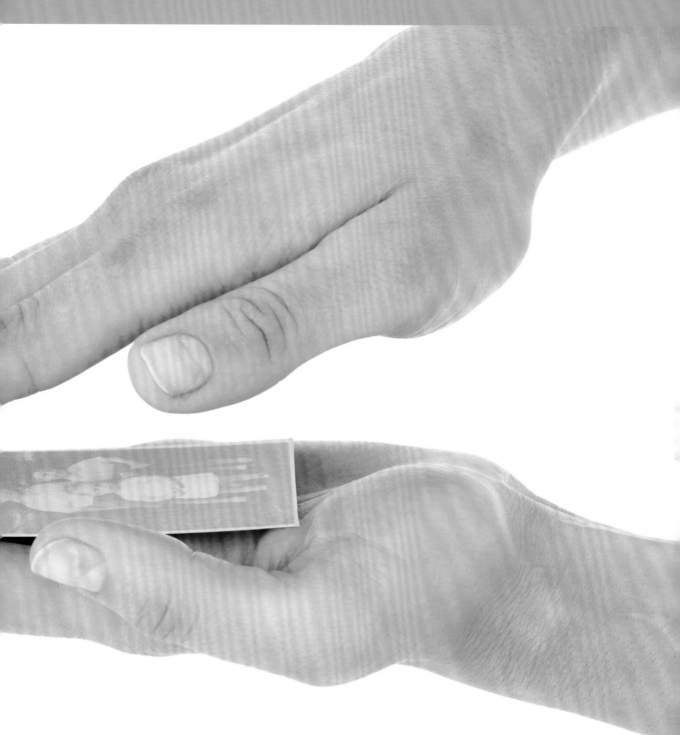

A photograph of a friend or family member can be used to focus your healing energy towards them, even if they are far away from you.

Distant Healing treatment

During Distant Healing, the healing power is amplified and the energy can be much stronger than during normal Reiki treatment, because mental forces are very vibrant. At the beginning of your treatment, always ask the receiver, mentally, whether they want to receive a healing from you; then wait for the answer to come. Never carry out a treatment against someone's will. The best way is to wait until you are asked for a Distant Healing.

Preparation

Before sending Distant Healing, make an appointment with the receiver. It is best if they are in a relaxed mood, either sitting or lying down. It will not affect the healing if they are active, but they are less likely to notice any physical, mental or emotional reactions. Distant Healing should not be sent to anyone undergoing an operation, since it can undermine the effects of the anaesthetic. However, it can be used safely both in preparation for the operation and to help healing afterwards. Do not send Reiki when someone is driving a car or operating machinery. Reiki often relaxes people so much that it can slow down their physical reactions.

Technique

The Distant Healing technique uses a form of visualization where your hands are in the same position and you visualize the person moving up and down or turning around. If you do not know the receiver personally, get a photo of them, or use a piece of paper and write their name and address on it. During the healing, you will notice where energy is absorbed most and which part of the body needs more Reiki. Spend a little extra time in these areas, either during or at the end of your treatment. Total treatment time varies from 20–30 minutes.

Instructions

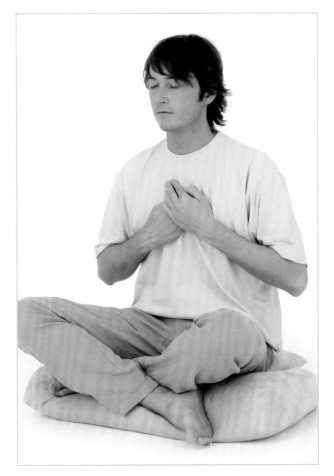

1 Sit comfortably, relax and centre yourself. Place your hands on your fourth (heart) chakra and meditate for a short while.

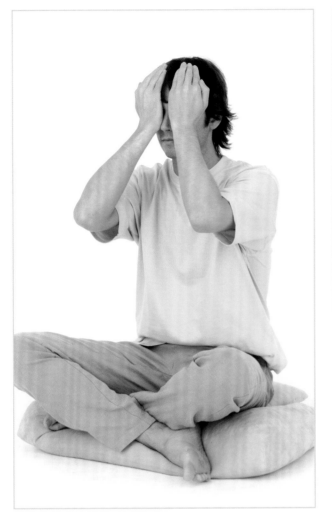

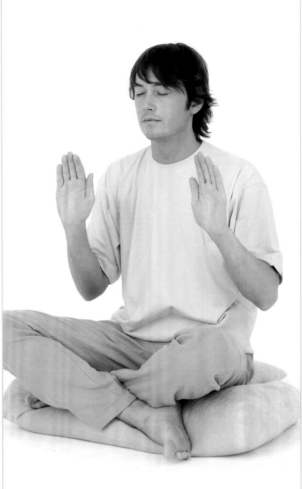

2 If you wish, give a little Reiki to your eyes, as in Head Position One (see page 128).

3 Invite the receiver to come and 'sit' in front of you. 'See' or 'feel' their presence, and ask if they want to receive a healing from you. Wait for the answer. If necessary, use the Power Symbol to bring the person to you. If the answer is 'Yes', continue with the healing (you will probably already have made an appointment for this). If you receive 'No', accept this and do not continue.

4 Visualize the receiver's forehead enlarged, raise your hands and draw the Distance Symbol, then draw the Power Symbol on top of it, to add more power.

5 Keeping your hands raised, visualize the symbols in golden light, repeat their names (the mantras) three times and repeat the receiver's name three times. Now say, 'I am sending you this healing energy in love. You can use it now or at any appropriate time.'

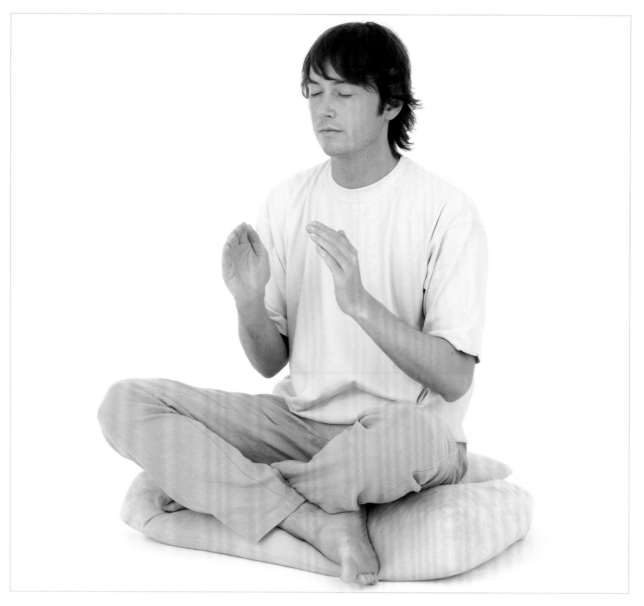

6 Sit comfortably, check whether the person is 'really there' and visualize their head at its normal size. 'Put' your hands on either side of the head and pull it towards you. Hold your hands in this position for about 3 minutes and give Reiki.

7 Now imagine the person is sitting in front of you, with their chest at the height of your hands. Draw a big Power Symbol on their chest and place your hands there for about 3 minutes.

8 Draw a Power Symbol on their abdomen area, and place your hands on it for about 3 minutes.

9 Now treat the receiver's back and ask the person to turn round. Draw a Power Symbol on their upper back, placing your hands there for about 3 minutes.

10 Draw a Power Symbol on their lower back, then place your hands there for about 3 minutes.

11 At the end, ask the person to turn round again and sit in front of you. Ask them how they feel and whether you can do anything else for them. Wait for a response.

12 Thank the person for receiving the healing and say goodbye. Rub your hands to break the connection with the Reiki symbols.

Healing old wounds

You can either use this form of healing on its own or integrate it into the normal Distant Healing treatment. When using it on its own, start with Steps 1–4 of Distant Healing (see instructions on pages 96–97), then continue directly with the instructions given below. When you integrate it into a standard Distant Healing treatment, complete Steps 1–10 of Distant Healing (see pages 96–98), then continue with the steps given below.

Instructions

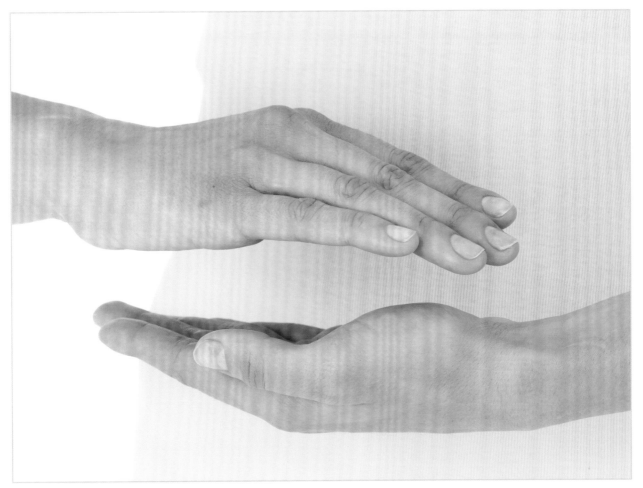

1 Visualize the receiver becoming very small, in the foetal position, between the palms of your hands.

2 Now draw the Harmony Symbol over their whole body, and then the Power Symbol on top of it, to add more power. Mentally give them the intention, or message, to let them 'do whatever they want'. This gives them permission to do what their heart desires, and not hold back any more. This can be a profound healing on the emotions and induces a healing of old wounds. Hold your hands until you feel the process is completed, for 5–10 minutes.

3 Ask the receiver to sit in front of you, and visualize them at their normal size again. Ask how they feel and if you can do anything else for them, and then wait.

4 Thank them for receiving the healing and say goodbye. At the end, rub your hands to break the connection with the Reiki symbols.

Permanent Distant Healing

This is a way of giving permanent healing to yourself or to another. You can give healing simultaneously to several themes, people, problem areas or health issues by using the Reiki Healing Box.

Healing Box

First, find a small wooden or cardboard box with a lid (don't use a metal box). With the Healing Box, you use all three symbols to send amplified healing energy (on all levels) to a person or an ongoing issue, such as an unresolved theme from childhood or any other current problem situation, related to work, a relationship or health. When sending healing to past events, such as difficult phases in your life, use a photo from the time you want to be healed. If you do not know the person in question, try to have a photo of them and write their name and address on the back. (This form of healing also works without a photo, but still write their name and address down.) Write each theme of the healing on a separate piece of paper and charge it with healing energy using all three Reiki symbols. Put as many issues as you like in the box at once.

Instructions

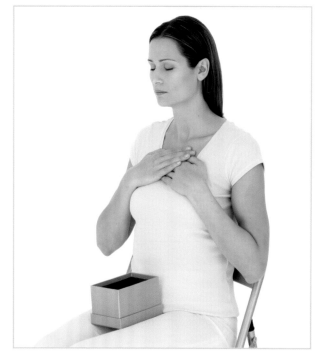

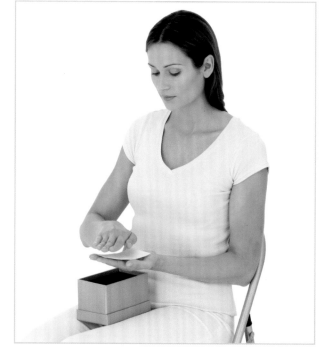

1 Sit comfortably and place your hands on your fourth chakra, bringing your awareness to your heart, preparing yourself by meditating for a short while.

2 Take the theme (written on a piece of paper) or the photo in your hands. Now 'draw' all three symbols on each theme or photo: the Distance Symbol to connect with the person or issue, the Harmony Symbol to reach all layers and the Power Symbol to empower the other two symbols.

3 Repeat all the mantras (the symbols' names) three times, visualizing them on the paper or photo, and repeat the receiver's name or theme of the healing three times.

4 Then repeat an invocation, such as the following: 'We are asking the universal life force, empowered by these active symbols, to shower its light, love and energy onto this person or issue now, and for as long as it is needed, for the highest good of everyone involved. We are grateful for these blessings.'

5 Repeat this sentence three times and check that all the symbols are still active. If necessary, visualize them again.

'We are asking the universal life force, empowered by these active symbols, to shower its light, love and energy onto this person or issue now, and for as long as it is needed, for the highest good of everyone involved.'

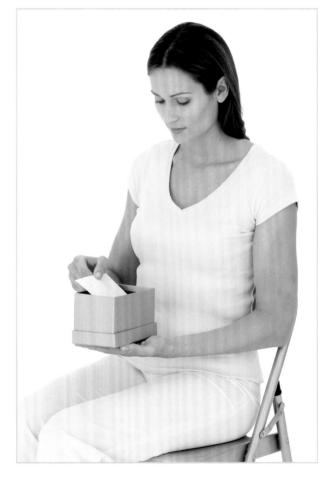

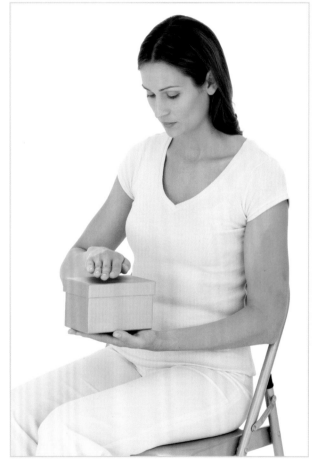

6 Treat each theme and each person individually and put it in the box. Go through the whole procedure for each issue. After dropping in each piece of paper or photo, rub your hands to break the connection with the Reiki symbols.

7 Then take the Healing Box in your hands and perform the whole procedure again on the entire box. Rub your hands together to break the connection. Then, once a day, carry out healing on the whole Healing Box for seven days. After that, reconsider each theme once more and renew each issue you wish to continue healing. If it is for another person, ask them if they wish to continue.

How to use the Second Degree

The tools of the Second Degree open up various possibilities for sending healing to past, present or future events via Distant Healing. In addition, you can work with deep-seated emotional issues via Mental Healing and concentrate on any difficult situation that needs attention. This means incorporating the two methods.

Mental Healing during Distant Healing

It is essential that you have the receiver's permission before embarking on Mental Healing via the Distant Healing technique.

Instructions

1 Start Distant Healing by using the Distance and Power symbols. Carry out the healing from Steps 1–5 (see pages 96–97).

2 Visualize with your inner eye (sixth chakra) and ask the person to lay down. Draw the Mental Healing symbols (Harmony and Power) above the head (crown chakra). Go through the procedure from Steps 4–14 of Mental Healing in your visualization (see page 89). Keep your eyes closed throughout.

3 Ask the receiver to sit again, visualize them at normal size and ask how they feel. Wait. Thank them for receiving the healing, say goodbye and rub your hands to break the connection.

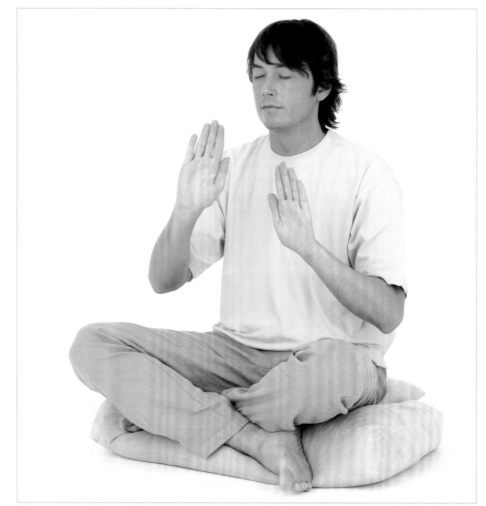

Mental Healing to a deceased person

You can give the Mental Healing to a deceased person to provide closure for yourself. Call them with the Distance Symbol and then put the Harmony Symbol between yourself and them. You are now connected at a higher level and can communicate from each other's Higher Self.

Mental Healing for deep emotional issues

Use Mental Healing to work with deep-seated emotions, such as fears, belief systems, habits (for instance, overeating), addictions (such as alcoholism), conditioning and childhood issues. Use both the Power Symbol and the Harmony Symbol.

Distant healing to ongoing issues in life

You can give Distant Healing to houses, crystals, businesses, ongoing life issues (work, a health problem, a relationship) by communicating from the Higher Self with the partner in question, using all three symbols.

Distant Healing to past events

You can work on themes going back into the distant past, such as traumatic events in childhood, to heal old wounds. Use a photo from that time, or write the problem down and ask Reiki to go to the cause of it. Use all three symbols when using a photo. Let the Reiki energy flow for 15 minutes, sensing the healing going to the hurt and being available to receive any insights from that time.

Distant Healing to future events

You can send Distant Healing 'on delivery' to future events, such as dental checks and operations. With your inner eye, visualize writing a label with a heading. Give exact details of the time and place when the healing should be received. Use all three symbols.

Distant healing for a dying friend

You can send Distant Healing to a dying friend or relative to bring relaxation, awareness and light, and perhaps your final goodbye. It works on all levels – physical, emotional, mental and spiritual – and can therefore heal old wounds and bring peace to all. Use all three symbols.

Distant Healing with animals

Use the Distant Healing technique and send Reiki to any animal at a distance. This is helpful when an animal might prove dangerous – for example, with animals in zoos or shelters – or when it may not be possible to touch an animal. Use the Distance Symbol and then add more power by using the Power Symbol on top. Or, if you wish, use all three symbols.

ADVICE FOR SENDING MENTAL AND DISTANT HEALING

- If possible, make an appointment with the receiver of Distant Healing, so that they know when the healing is to be sent.
- If you have not arranged a specific time, ask the receiver, at the beginning of the healing contact, whether they want to receive healing from you.
- Don't give Reiki during surgery, as it can disturb the effectiveness of anaesthetic. Make a label (see below left) to deliver healing after surgery has been completed.
- If you notice your own thoughts and judgements bubbling up during the healing, tell the receiver to ignore them, and apologize. Try to keep your mind as empty as possible.
- Be aware of so-called 'helper-trips' – when it feels good to help others – rendering your motives suspect. It is usually good to wait until you are asked for healing rather than offer it.
- Give yourself Mental and Distant Healing, and find things out for yourself, at any time. This supports your personal process and healing.

Distant Healing to treat your garden

Using the Distant Healing method to treat your garden can be very effective and may enable it to flourish. If you have a drawn plan showing all the various features, you can give Distant Healing to the plan, or visualize the trees and plants in good condition, growing healthily. Use the Distance Symbol, then add more power by using the Power Symbol on top.

'The Second Degree training was excellent and a big step forward for me. Learning the Distant Healing and Mental Healing, I felt great peace. I found the whole weekend very enlightening and am keen to use Reiki in my hospital work.'

Ben

Sending Distant Healing to the planet

We are all responsible for what happens on earth and need to wake up to help our planet survive. There are many ways in which we can support and evoke positive energies for contributing awareness, intelligence, love and healing to world situations. Reiki is a powerful gift that we can use for this purpose. In times of general unrest, during disasters and wars, you can send Reiki to the whole earth, or concentrate on specific regions. This can include natural catastrophes, conflicts between religious groups, countries and people.

Group Reiki

Because Reiki energy is stronger in a group, get together with Reiki friends and let thoughts of peace, love and healing energy flow to the whole planet or specific areas that are in difficulty. Use the Distant Group Healing method (see pages 102–103) or the Reiki Healing Box (see pages 100–101).

Instructions

1 Write down the name of the place or situation and hold the piece of paper.

2 Trace the Distance Symbol, then the Harmony Symbol and then the Power Symbol on top, repeating all their mantras three times.

3 Give the intention that Reiki should go to that situation 'for the highest good' for all involved. In this way, Reiki includes all aspects of the situation and includes the entire picture, such as the people who live there, their governments, aid agencies, warring factions and so on.

WORLD HEALING MEDITATION

The world healing meditation happens on the last day of each month and on 31 December annually; it is sent at 12 noon (Greenwich Mean Time/13.00 MET/Middle European Time). The first time this meditation happened was on 31 December 1986, when more than 41 million people participated. Try sending healing energy on a mental level, using the Distant Healing method, to the whole earth or specific areas in need. Imagine holding the whole globe between your hands and send it Reiki. Use the Distance Symbol to connect you to the earth and the Power Symbol to give it more power.

Earth healing

You can give Reiki to power centres and sacred places. If you are physically present at these ancient spots, visualize a huge Power Symbol over the top of the area. You can either sit in the middle of the place or put your hands on part of the building, structure or object. Let Reiki energy flow around, then allow it to flow into the earth itself. Another way to give healing to the earth is by sitting or standing (outdoors or indoors) and drawing a huge Power Symbol over the earth or floor. Direct the Reiki energy into the earth with your palms facing downwards.

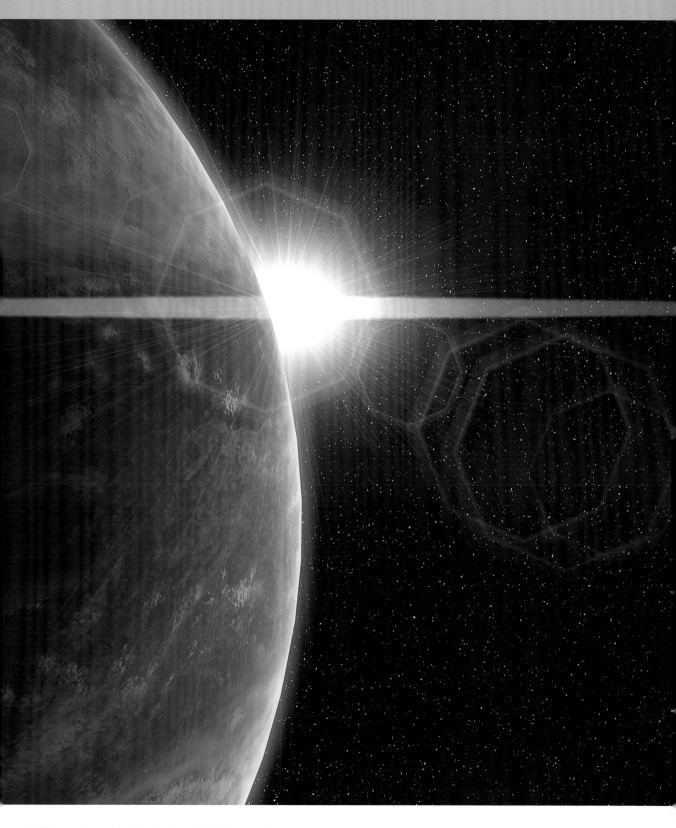

Reiki can be sent to the whole earth to help our planet
survive. Try Group Reiki or world healing meditation to send
positive, healing energy to areas of the world with difficulties.

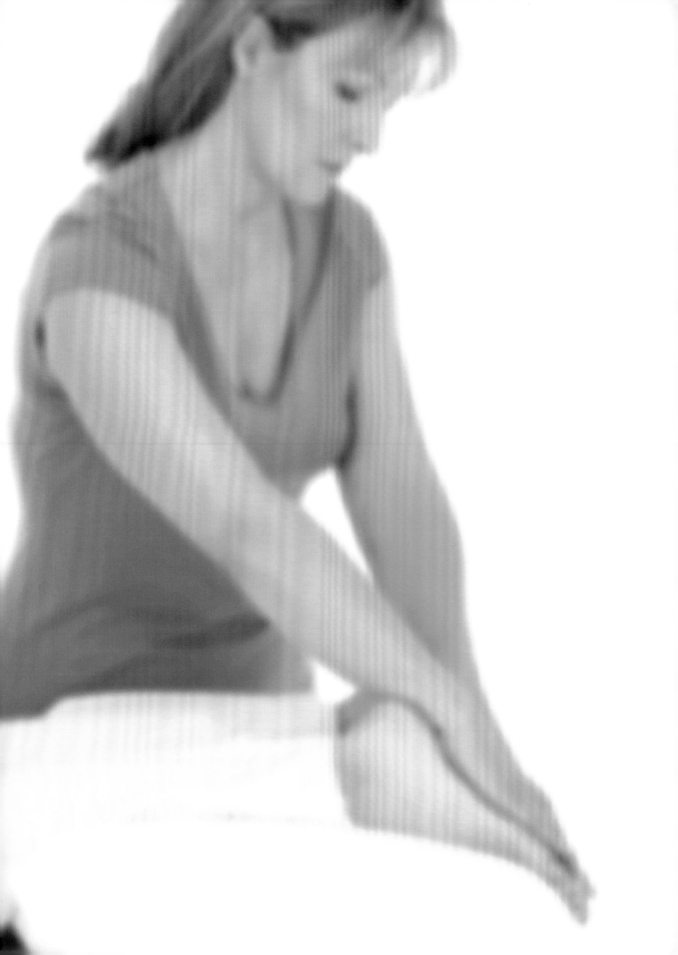

The Third Degree

The Third Degree expands the flow of Reiki energy and deepens each student's healing. It lifts personal energy and consciousness to a far higher level of awareness than before. It is for personal development, and interacts with all aspects of life. You have to 'live' Reiki; it is a life commitment to a healing practice and a spiritual discipline. This degree, in which the student becomes a qualified Master-Teacher of Reiki, is for those who have sufficient experience and feel a vocation to give and receive healing.

Preparing for the Third Degree

'Why do you want to become a Reiki Master-Teacher?' This is the question all Third Degree candidates have to answer. It is important to explore your motivation, as this helps you decide whether you are ready for this next step. Most students sense a desire to share the gift of Reiki; it feels 'right' to do the Third Degree. Reiki has already become part of life, and it is a privilege to feel the desire to pass on that experience. If you love Reiki and are aware of the responsibility of what it means to be a Reiki Master, then it is the right time to become one.

The role of the Master

As a Master, you have to commit to bearing responsibility; you recognize that you yourself are 'master' of your life. In the process of becoming a Reiki Master, you have to investigate and challenge old, perhaps negative thought patterns, attitudes and behaviours, replacing them with more life-affirming and positive ones. The Third Degree requires you to take a big step forward in life. The attunement to the Third Degree triggers profound development and gives you the opportunity for substantial personal growth on all levels: physical, mental, emotional and spiritual.

Realizing the Self

To truly be a Master, you need to realize your own real 'Self' and recognize 'who you are': a divine being of love and light. True Mastery means to live in a state of light, wisdom and knowing. You have moved beyond personality and negative beliefs; the struggling of the 'ego' can stop. You can start simply enjoying life for what it is. You begin loving and respecting yourself just as you are; perfect the way you are. Reiki is a great gift and guides you on your path towards realization and enlightenment, returning 'home', knowing your essence and 'who you really are'.

A tool for awakening

Being a Reiki Master-Teacher is not just about how to initiate others into Reiki and how to teach it; it is more than a healing method – it is a spiritual discipline and a wonderful tool that you can use for your own awakening. You need more than knowledge and practical experience; you need self-awareness, understanding, wisdom, compassion and a love for life and others; you need skill in supporting students in their own personal, spiritual journey towards self-realization. The role of a Reiki Master is that of a respected teacher ('Sensei' in Japanese); someone for whom Reiki is an essential part of daily life. For each Master, Reiki is a very personal journey, because each person comes from a different starting point, with a unique story, which finally brought them to Reiki. When you are attuned to the Reiki power, you have Reiki for life; and when you become a Master, Reiki becomes your whole life.

Blocked energy flow

An important key in healing is when we become aware that our feelings are cut off from energy. In the body this causes an energy 'block'. Now we can become aware of how we have misunderstood life and know what lessons we need to learn. This energy-flow disturbance is connected with our feelings of separation from the Divine and needs to be reconnected through the use of Reiki.

Higher energy

Because the Reiki healing system uses energy-transmission to raise the vibratory rate of our physical and energy bodies, we are able to let a higher energy force flow through us. This not only affects us, but also our surroundings, and actually heightens the vibratory rate of the earth itself.

The role of Reiki Master-Teacher means more than initiating others into the healing method – it demands a high level of spiritual maturity and a major life commitment.

Preparing to become a Master

As soon as a student has booked the Third Degree training, the process of becoming a Master starts. As a practical preparation, each Master student should have a Reiki self-treatment every day, even if it is just for 15 minutes in the morning or evening.

Raised levels of vibration

During the weeks leading up to the Master training, it is vital to raise the vibrational frequency of your energy bodies on all levels. During the last two weeks before the training, it is recommended that you do a full daily self-treatment. This gives your energy system good preparation for the power that will be coming through you. These treatments can be done as exchange treatments with other Reiki friends or practitioners, increasing and clearing the flow of energy and loosening any blockages.

Daily meditation practice

It is also beneficial to meditate more often, preferably every day. Just sit silently and watch your breath (or practise your usual meditation method), or meditate on the Reiki symbols and principles. Contemplate your motives for becoming a Reiki Master and the responsibilities and commitment that they imply.

In preparation for the Master training, it is advisable to have a Reiki self-treatment every day, as well as to meditate on a more frequent basis.

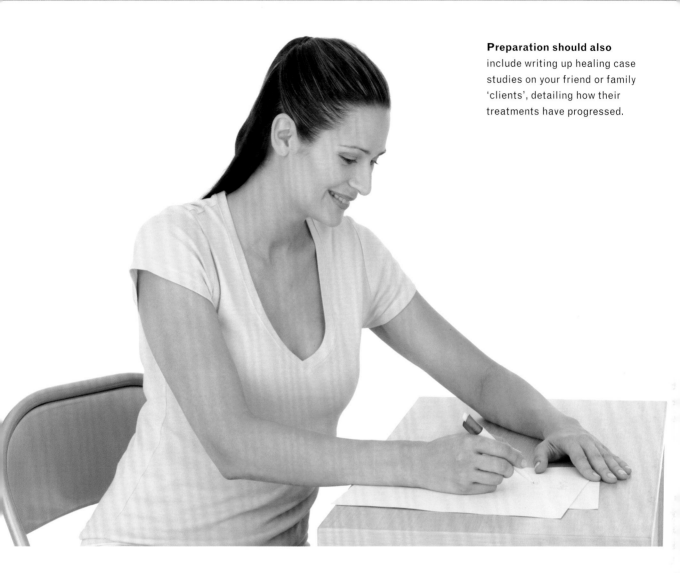

Preparation should also include writing up healing case studies on your friend or family 'clients', detailing how their treatments have progressed.

Further studies

Also look at yourself and all the experiences you already have. You might decide that you want to attend a personal-growth seminar for clearing personal issues. To increase your self-confidence before becoming a Reiki teacher, perhaps you could acquire a teaching qualification or gain some experience in some form of teaching (especially if you are not familiar with this). Inspiring reading material, especially on spiritual matters, as recommended by your Reiki Master, can be a useful support, connecting you more deeply with yourself and with Reiki, and preparing you for the Master training on a spiritual and energetic level.

Case studies

It is very helpful for each student to write reports (in the form of healing case studies) on at least two Reiki 'clients',

who can be friends or family members. These studies represent between four and six treatments per client. Make notes after giving each Reiki treatment about what you noticed and how the treatment is progressing. This will help you to become aware of any changes that Reiki healing brings about.

'It [Reiki] is an art of living and healing. Any art requires discipline – the discipline of faith, commitment, focus and self-control.'

Paul Mitchell, Office of Reiki Grand Master, talking about 'Discipline and the Usui System'

The attunement process

Reiki Masters are ordinary human beings who know that they are masters of their own lives. The Master Degree takes you a step forward in life, but becoming a Master does not come automatically through being attuned. You need to be committed to Reiki and accept the challenge for your own personal development. This brings changes to many aspects of your life.

Single attunement

There is a single attunement during the Third Degree. This takes place during a sacred ceremony and is an essential part of the Master training. It heightens the vibratory frequency and activates the energy of the Master Symbol. One of the most important aspects of the Master training is the complex process of stimulating and activating energy-transmission ('attunement' or 'initiation') with all the associated Reiki symbols. A fully initiated Master activates the higher vibration of the Master Symbol and can direct the force of the symbol for work with others, to open their channel for Reiki energy. The energy of Reiki and the activated symbols is transmitted to the student's mind, body and spirit. Afterwards, whenever the student uses the symbols, the same energy they received during attunement is activated and begins to flow.

Cleansing process

Being initiated into the Third Degree is a powerful spiritual experience. It touches the student deeply on all levels: physical, mental, emotional and spiritual. The Master Symbol has a strong vibration and enters the consciousness directly, to bring light to the receiver. The attunement makes the student a wide channel for Universal Life Energy to flow through. This is experienced differently by each student (see pages 66–67). Each attunement triggers a form of cleansing, which is normal because the body and its energy system first need to adjust to the higher frequency and vibrational energy (see the 21-Day Cleansing Process, page 76).

Energetic connection

The Master initiation creates an energetic connection between Reiki Master and newly initiated Master, as both are part of the direct Reiki lineage going back to the source of Reiki. All Masters call upon this when initiating others into Reiki.

There is considerable variation in the quality, style and content of the Master-Teacher training among Reiki Masters of the present day. However, it is common to be taught the Master training over a short period of time, between 1–10 days, usually over 1–6 months, although some Reiki Masters teach the Third Degree over a three-day period.

Training structure

In the early days of Reiki in the West (during the early 1990s), Reiki Masters (especially members of the Reiki Alliance) were taught via an apprenticeship system, where a Master student worked alongside a fully experienced Master-Teacher for a year. This involved learning how to organize and teach First and Second Degree classes through observation, sometimes taking over certain parts of the teaching to gain experience and confidence. Over time, when the Master considered that the student was ready, the student was given the Master Symbol, received the Master attunement and learnt all the initiation rituals for the attunements of the First and Second Degrees. How to attune to the Third Degree was frequently not taught until several years later, when the newly qualified Reiki Master had gained plenty of additional experience.

It is recommended that all students find a training structure that leaves plenty of time and opportunity for experiencing Reiki on all the various levels. The Master training should be designed to give the opportunity to train as a Master, while receiving all the knowledge and expertise to become a fully initiated Reiki Master of the Usui system.

Degree content

The Third Degree training includes revising the teachings of the First and Second Degrees and undergoing teaching observation. This means that you review your knowledge about the hand positions (see page 126) and Mental and Distant Healing practices (see pages 86 and 96). Part of the teaching is to transmit a deep knowledge about the four Reiki symbols: their qualities, significance and use (see page 79). It is also important to re-examine your Reiki practice, and for you to receive supervision and feedback on specific cases. There are meetings between you and your Master to clarify questions concerning practice, the Mastery process and personal issues. These meetings focus on whatever is most important to you, and treatments are exchanged between you and the Master.

Usually the final teaching is conveyed over three consecutive days. You receive the teaching of the Master Symbol and are instructed how to use it (see page 116). All the initiation rituals of First, Second and Third Degrees are taught, and there is plenty of time to practise the attunement methods of all three degrees. There is discussion on spiritual and business responsibilities as a Reiki Master, and guidelines are given for teaching practice, such as when to start training others, the form a class should take, and issues such as training fees. The Master attunement and the empowerment with the Master Symbol are given at the very end of the training.

After a Reiki Master training

Being attuned as a Reiki Master is the beginning of a long journey towards 'Mastery'. At this level, spiritual development is a key part of your life. Reiki guides you towards spiritual awakening, which gives you greater love, wisdom and understanding about yourself and others. As for the First and Second Degrees, you go though a 21-day cleansing process, but the effects may be deeper, as the Master attunement has a higher vibration.

You might not want to attune anyone else for a month or two after you have become a Master. Instead, use the Master Symbol (see Meditation with the Master Symbol, page 119) and its higher energies for personal healing and spiritual development. Use the symbols in your self-treatment and on others. Only start initiating others when you feel that it is the right time for you. Trust your intuition in this matter. Some newly initiated Masters let several years lapse before they feel that the time is right.

By becoming a Reiki Master, you are taking one significant step forward in your spiritual journey, which brings changes to many aspects of your life.

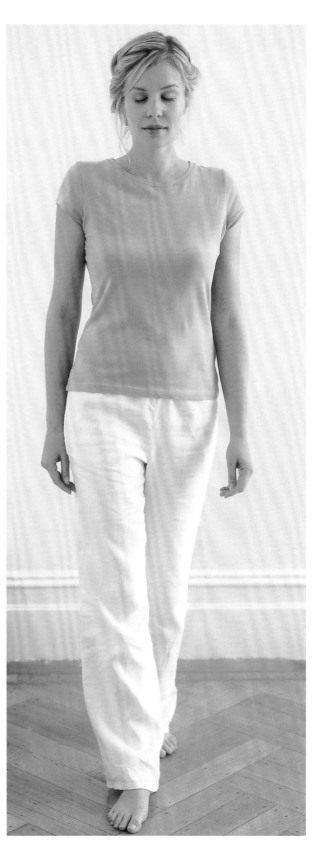

The Master Symbol

The Master Symbol is the Fourth Symbol, which comes from Kanji, the Japanese writing system, and consists of 19 strokes. It describes the Buddha nature, our true essence, in which we become aware of what we really are. We experience enlightenment, or 'satori'.

Meaning

The symbol's mantra means 'great light' or 'great enlightenment'. The Master Symbol admits higher and purer dimensions of light and healing, and assists you in accessing intuition and a deep understanding of your true being. It is connected with the seventh chakra. The Master Symbol can be used alone, usually for meditation and purification, and in combination with the other symbols during the attunement process. It thus increases their effectiveness and enables them to work using only their purest intention. Using the Master Symbol will affect your spiritual development. In this way, Reiki becomes a vehicle on the path to personal perfection.

Purpose of the Master Symbol

The main function of the symbol is to raise your level of consciousness and to open yourself as a pure channel. It awakens a strong force and initiates a vibration to open the channel of others and yourself for higher energies. When using the symbol, you create a direct connection to the light, the source, within. You automatically connect with the Higher Self and the awakened part of your being, which is full of wisdom. The symbol is intended for meditation and refines your energies for your own awakening. If you meditate with the symbol on a regular basis, it opens you to become a wider and purer channel to let Reiki flow through you and access Reiki healing.

THE IMPORTANCE OF MATURITY

Before Hawayo Takata died, she authorized her granddaughter Phyllis Lei Furumoto to initiate Reiki students into the Master's Degree. In 1988, Grand Master Furumoto granted authorization for all Reiki Masters who felt matured through personal Reiki practice to attune others into the Master Degree. Traditional Usui Masters recommend waiting a minimum of five years before training as a Reiki Master, but as a consequence of this rule relaxation, there are now many Masters who failed to receive proper, simple Reiki because they were initiated by Masters who were too new to the discipline. This created a situation whereby today there are Masters who are 20 generations old (in Reiki lineage) in just five years. They have missed out on simple teaching and maturation, which takes time, experience and patience.

It is important for all newly initiated Reiki Masters to have plenty of experience with the First and Second Degree classes before initiating other students into Reiki Mastery. As a Master, you need to be energetically ready and to have had plenty of teaching practice before taking responsibility for guiding a Master student. It is recommended that you have a minimum of three years' practice as an active Reiki Master before initiating other Masters.

Remember that Hawayo Takata practised for 35 years before initiating her first Master. Her teaching was simple, and the clarity and discipline of her practice gave this simplicity its power. Her knowledge became 'knowing', which came from her Reiki-Teacher and was confirmed by many years of practice. This is the discipline and the sense of really 'knowing' this healing art, which comes from years of trust and experience.

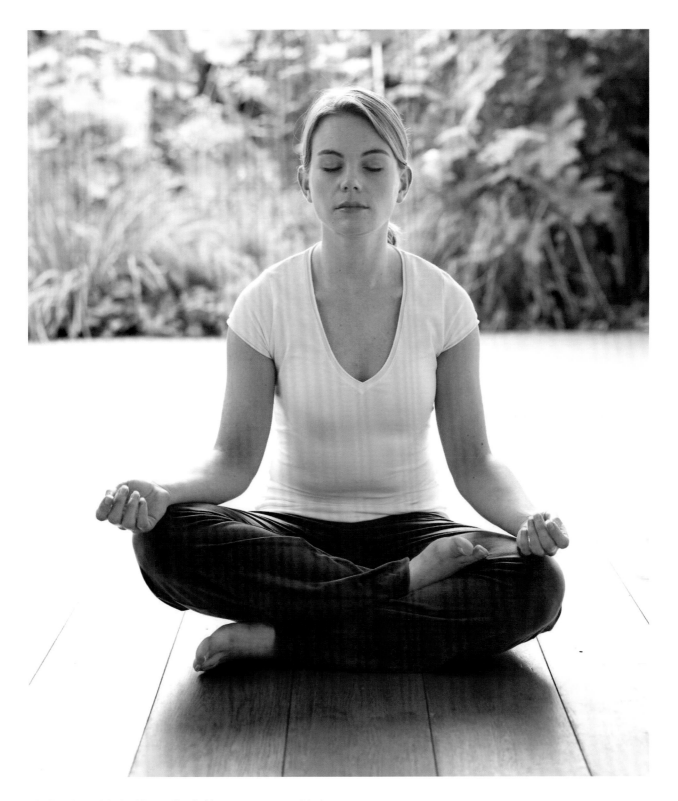

Meditating with the Master Symbol lets you connect with the
Higher Self – the wise part in you – which will support you in
your personal growth and work with others.

Uses of the Master Symbol

The Master Symbol is a very strong force and is used by the Master to channel higher energies during attunement. In addition, you can use it to surround yourself with its higher and 'finer' vibrations, to create harmony and balance. Because the Master Symbol vibrates at a higher frequency, it can connect you at a deep level with your Higher Consciousness and bring you into higher dimensions; to the Source of All. This can give you valuable insights into life and its purpose.

When working with the Master Symbol, 'draw' it in the same way as the other symbols, with the whole hand (or the fingers of one hand), visualize it in bright or golden light and say its mantra three times. Here are eight ways in which you can use the Master Symbol.

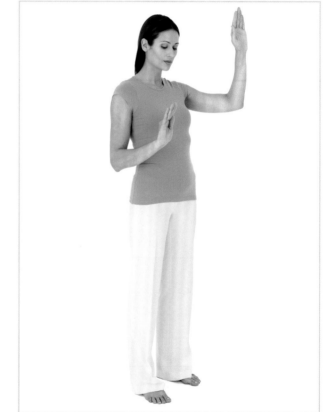

Instructions

1 Visualize the Master Symbol in a white or golden light. Also experiment with other colours, such as purple, violet, pink, turquoise or rainbow colours, and see how this influences you.

2 Visualize the Master Symbol and hold the image in your mind to meditate upon. Repeat its mantra three times (in silence or out loud, if you are alone).

3 'Draw' the symbol in front of you and step into it: the symbol is multi-dimensional energy, with height, width and depth. Visualize it as filling your whole being.

4 Visualize the symbol in front of you and breathe it in with each in-breath. Then let the symbol fill your whole body.

5 'Draw' the Master Symbol in front of you, visualize it in golden light and chant its mantra (out loud, if you are alone) to purify and fill your body with its energy: light, love and peace. Do this before and after any activity.

6 Sit and meditate with the symbol, to give any problem or difficulty to Reiki in trust. The solution will come to you via your intuition. You can also use this method to infuse any world disaster with love, peace and healing.

7 Use the Master Symbol when giving yourself Mental Healing. Visualize it or 'draw' it on the back of your head and let it enter your whole body. Then continue with the normal procedure of Mental Healing (see pages 92–93).

8 Use the Master Symbol with the other symbols to create a safe, sacred space for initiation ceremonies.

Meditation with the Master Symbol

At Master level, you can activate and feel the vibration of the symbol, so to sit and meditate with it can bring great benefits. This has a strong, positive force and enters the consciousness directly, bringing light to the receiver. This has an effect on your physical, mental, emotional and spiritual levels, and the light can enter the darkest corners and loosen blockages on all planes. It is recommended for a Master to meditate using the symbol each day.

Instructions

1 Sit in a relaxed and comfortable posture (on a chair or on the floor). Keep your spine straight and your eyes closed.

2 (a) Imagine and 'draw' the Master Symbol from your inner eye (the sixth chakra) in front of you or over the top of your head (the seventh chakra). Visualize it in golden light and repeat its mantra three times.
(b) Alternatively, draw the Master Symbol with your hands raised in front of you, visualize it in golden light and repeat the mantra three times.

3 Allow the symbol to enter you and flow into your entire body. Feel the vibration of the symbol inside you, repeating the mantra (out loud, if you are alone).

4 Feel the energy and vibration that the symbol creates and notice how it affects you. Sit and meditate with the Master Symbol as long as you want to.

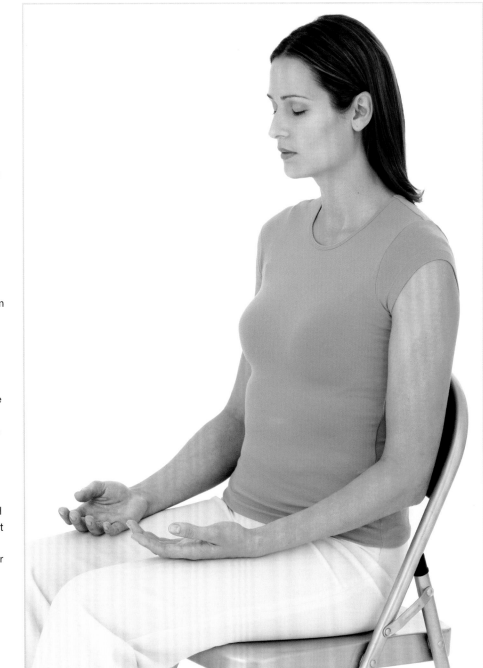

Learning how to attune others

Part of the Master training is to learn how to attune others into the Reiki method. How to stimulate an energy-transmission and activate higher energies to open up the 'inner healing channel' of a receiver is an important part of the training. This book contains only the theory and principles of attuning others, since this part of the training is confidential and is only passed on from Master to student.

Creating a sacred space

Each attunement is carried out in a sacred ceremony in a specially prepared space. Each Master has his or her own style of creating a sacred space, but it is recommended that you have a small altar with Usui's picture, some flowers, candles, perhaps incense and healing stones. The Master prepares this room energetically with the Reiki symbols in advance of the ceremony, to clear out old energies and bring in fresh, positive vibrations. Usually, the student is initiated either alone or in a small group of 2–4 people.

The initiation ceremony

The receiver's eyes are closed during the whole process of energy-transmission. The initiating Master repeats an invocation before the initiation, such as: 'Let yourself be touched by this Universal Life Energy, called Reiki, and let its love, light and energy shower on you.' The student raises his folded hands in the Gassho position (also called 'Namaste', the prayer position; see page 63) in front of the forehead. The Reiki Master starts the attunement from behind, by drawing the symbols over the top of the head (crown chakra), and channels the symbols into the receiver's body. Then the Master moves in front of the student, carries out an empowerment over the folded hands and continues with the remainder of the procedure. For the entire process, the Master works with each student individually, starting from the back, moving to the side and the front. The student feels some gentle contact and blowing on the head and hands. At the end, the student's entire aura is filled with the energy of a big Power Symbol. Then their hands are placed in their lap.

The First, Second and Third Degree attunements are similar – the main difference being when the actual empowerment with the Reiki symbols itself takes place.

The quality of the Reiki energy is the same in each attunement, but the quantity and vibration are different. Before and after the initiation it is recommended that each student has time to remain quiet and perhaps be on their own to contemplate the effects of the attunement. Being in silence, meditating, sitting or lying, or connecting with nature is very supportive.

Attuning other Masters

To be well prepared to attune others into the Master Degree and feel really ready for this next step, you, as a Master, must have practised Reiki, by giving treatments and teaching First and Second Degree classes, for several years. This is important, because the Reiki energy passing through you vibrates at a higher frequency and can be very strong, especially the first time you initiate a Reiki Master. To transmit this high vibration of energy can be like receiving an initiation yourself, again. The full measure of the power and force transmitted in an attunement depends on the development of the initiating Master and how much energy their physical body can hold. The spiritual development, integrity and correctness of the attunement rituals of an active Master are just as important as their knowledge and experience with Reiki.

'Let yourself be touched by this Universal Life Energy, called Reiki, and let its love, light and energy shower on you.'

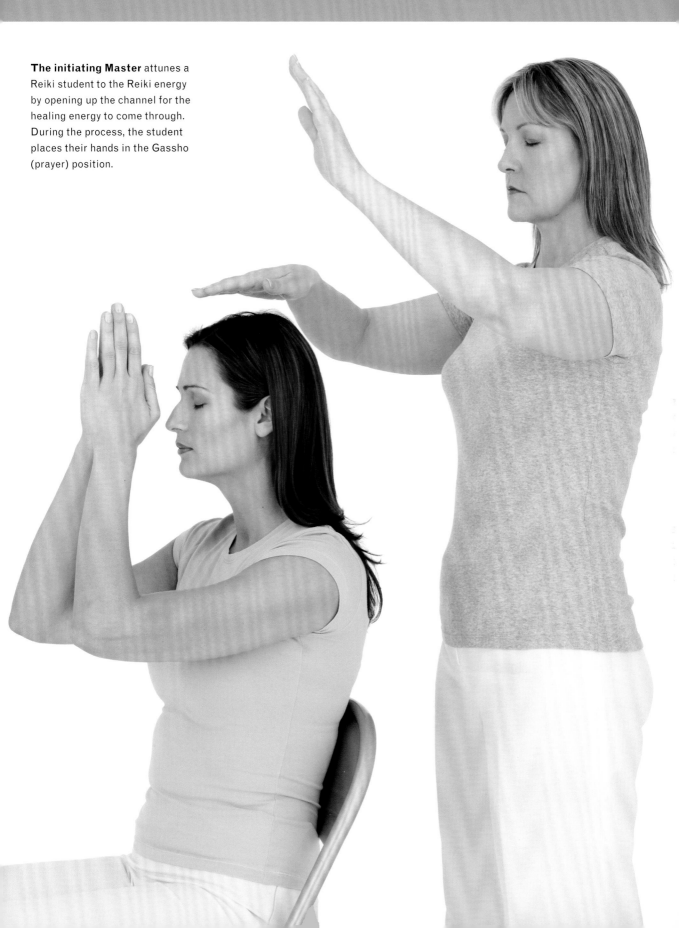

The initiating Master attunes a Reiki student to the Reiki energy by opening up the channel for the healing energy to come through. During the process, the student places their hands in the Gassho (prayer) position.

Advanced chakra balancing

To gain more experience with different forms of treatments within the Reiki method, you can use advanced chakra balancing. This will help you become more sensitive to the energy flow in the chakras and the energy bodies of another person (receiver). It will also enhance your intuition, sensitivity and trust in your own ability to sense energies.

Harmonizing the chakras

Because the basic Reiki positions follow the seven main chakras, you can integrate the harmonization of the chakras into a single Reiki treatment. You can also treat the energy centres separately. The process usually takes 15–20 minutes. Each chakra reflects an aspect of personal growth. If the chakra energy flow is blocked, this may lead to an imbalance and to mental, spiritual or physical disorder. With the help of Reiki, you can harmonize, or balance out, an excess or shortage of energy in your chakras. As a rule, there is often too much energy in the head and too little in the lower body. The seventh chakra does not need any additional energy, so do not touch it in the course of this treatment.

Let the hands rest on the two chakras that require balancing until you can feel the same energy in both. This usually takes 2–3 minutes. Sometimes you may feel a temperature difference between your hands, ranging from warm to cold, or experience other sensations, such as tingling in your hands. When you notice this, wait until you feel both hands becoming the same temperature. The treatment lasts for 20–30 minutes.

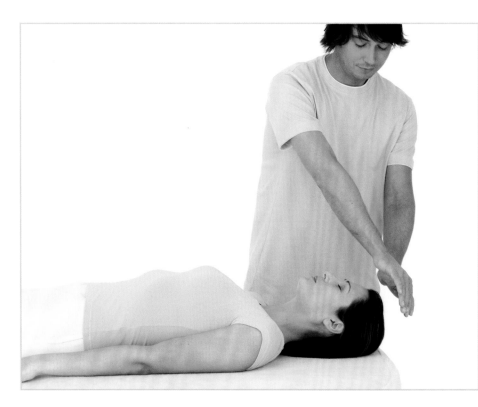

Smoothing the aura

Let the receiver lie on their back; the arms should be relaxed on either side. Smooth the receiver's aura from head to toe, using smooth, curving movements, starting at the head and working down to the feet. Do this three times. It has a relaxing effect on the receiver and prepares them for the treatment to come.

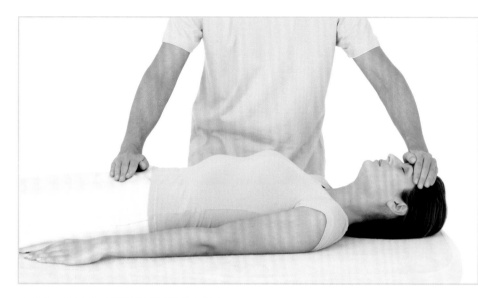

First and sixth chakras

Lay one hand on the first chakra and the other on the sixth chakra and keep them there until you can sense the same amount of energy flowing in both centres. When treating a woman, you can actually touch the pubic bone, but when treating a man you should hold your hand a short distance above the pubic area.

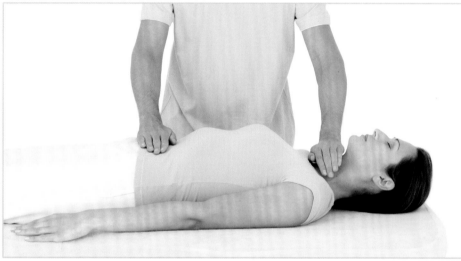

Second and fifth chakras

Lay one hand on the second chakra and the other just over the fifth chakra, but without actually touching the throat. Rest there until you sense balanced energy between the two centres.

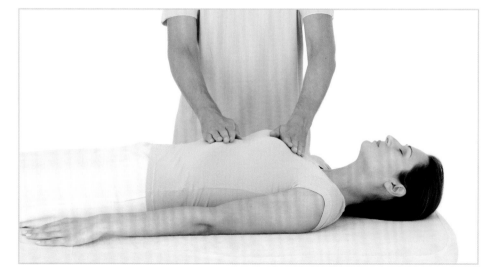

Third and fourth chakras

Lay one hand on the third chakra and the other on the fourth chakra. Rest there until you sense balanced energy between both centres.

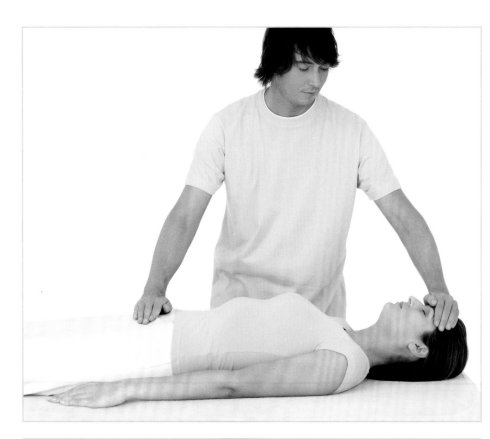

Emotional balancing

You can now deepen the healing with emotional balancing. Place one hand on the lower abdomen, just below the navel, and the other on the forehead. After a couple of minutes, move your hand clockwise in slow motion over the lower abdomen a few times. This creates deep relaxation for the receiver and helps him or her let go of thoughts, feelings and tensions in the body.

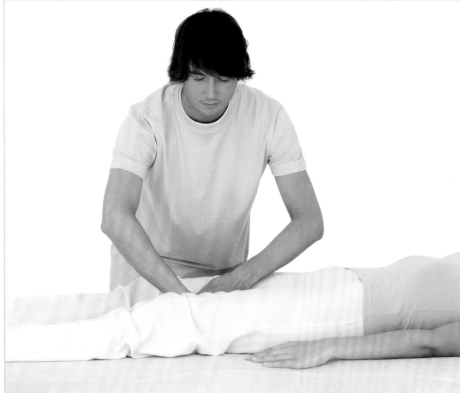

Releasing further tensions

To release further tensions, lay your hands flat on the insides of each thigh, between the upper legs (fingertips pointing in opposite directions). This helps the receiver let go of their fears, which are often held in the stomach or belly area.

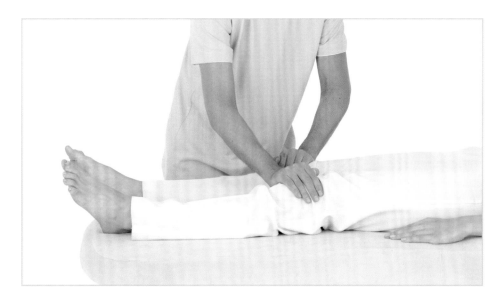

Releasing fears

Place each hand on one knee. By giving Reiki here you can release tension and fear, especially fear of moving forward in life or the fear of dying.

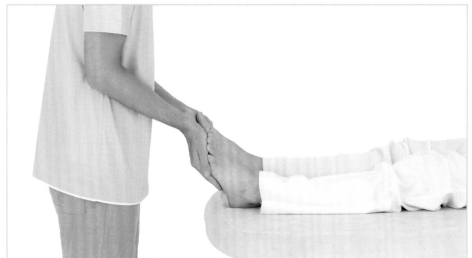

Grounding all the chakras

Rest the base of the palms of your hands on the toes and point your fingertips towards the heels. Or lay your hands on the soles of the feet, ideally with the fingertips covering the toes. This strengthens the root chakra and grounds all the chakras.

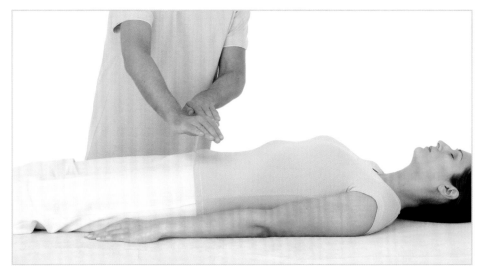

Resmoothing the aura

At the end of the treatments, smooth the aura again twice from head to toe, then draw an energy line from the pubic bone up over the head.

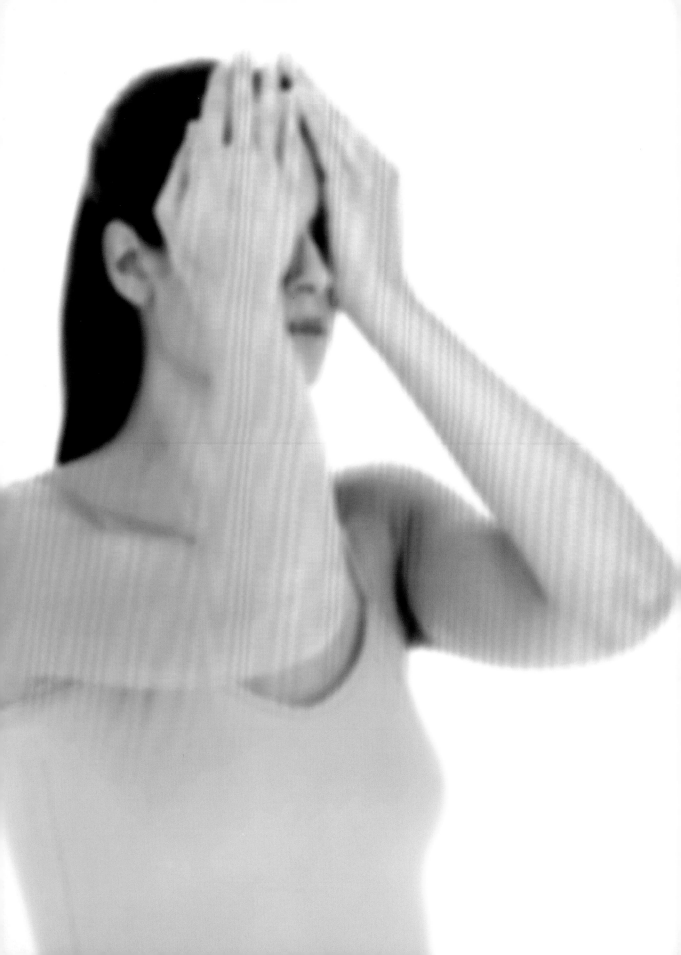

The Reiki hand positions

In this chapter you will find the basic Reiki hand positions, showing how to give a full-body Reiki treatment to yourself and to another person. The positions shown in this book cover all the main body organs, all the glands of the endocrine system, immune system, autonomous nervous system, the main meridians, the acupressure points and all the seven main chakras. There are additional hand positions that you can use to treat specific disturbances and imbalances in the body.

Self-treatment

Use the basic Reiki self-treatment sequence on yourself whenever you have the opportunity. When preparing for the Third Degree (see Chapter 5, page 108), it is advisable to practise this every day. It is a good idea to try to integrate self-treatment into your daily routine, such as 15–30 minutes in the morning and another 15–30 in the evening, or at any time of the day that suits you. When placing your hands on your own body, do not use pressure. Lay your hands gently and adjust them to your body's contours and shape.

The 15 self-treatment positions

Hold each hand position for 3–5 minutes, or longer if desired. If you wish, you can smooth your own aura at the beginning of the treatment. Move your hands along the body in a downward movement to calm the energy of the aura (see page 62).

Head Position One

Put your hands over your eyes, resting your palms on your cheekbones. This position helps colds, produces clarity of thought, aids stress reduction and intuition, and facilitates meditation.

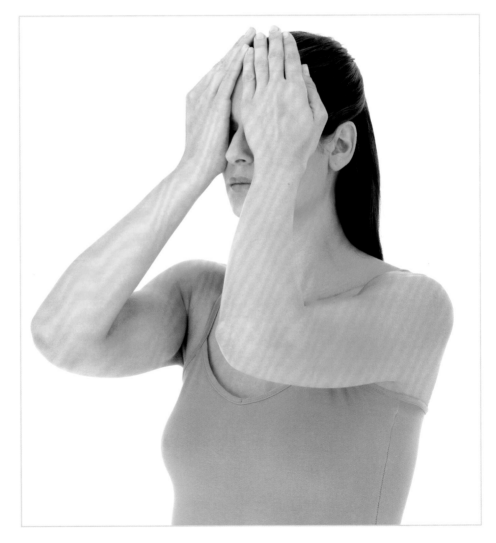

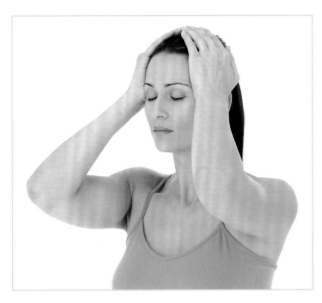

Head Position Two

Place your hands on either side of your head, above your ears, with the base of your palms touching your temples, the fingers following the curve of your head. This position harmonizes the two sides of the brain, and improves memory and the enjoyment of life. It is helpful for depression and headaches.

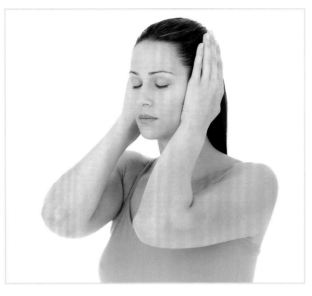

Head Position Three

Place your hands on either side of your head, covering your ears. This comforting position affects the entire body. It is helpful for earache and eases the symptoms of colds and flu.

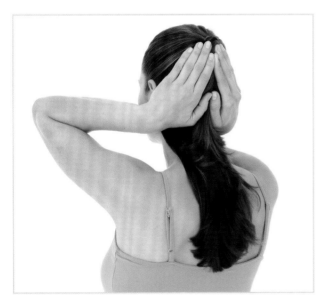

Head Position Four

Place your hands on the back of your head, holding your head like a ball, fingers pointing upwards. This position eases sleep disorders, conveys a sense of security, promotes intuition, helps headaches, relieves fears and depression, and calms the mind and the emotions.

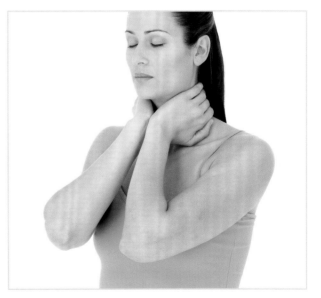

Head Position Five

Place your hands around your throat, with your wrists touching in the centre. This position harmonizes blood pressure and metabolism, helps neck pains and hoarseness, and promotes self-expression.

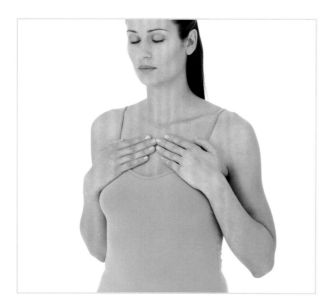

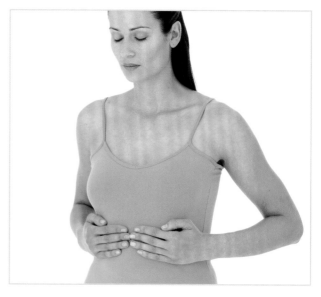

Front Position One

Place your hands on either side of your upper chest, fingers touching, just below the collarbone. This position strengthens the immune system, regulates heart and blood pressure, stimulates lymph circulation, increases the capacity for love and enjoyment of life, and transforms negativity.

Front Position Two

Place your hands over your lower ribcage, above the waist, fingers touching in the middle. This position regulates the digestion, gives energy, promotes relaxation, and reduces fears and frustration.

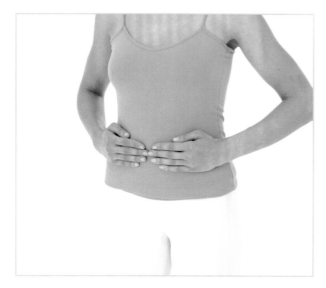

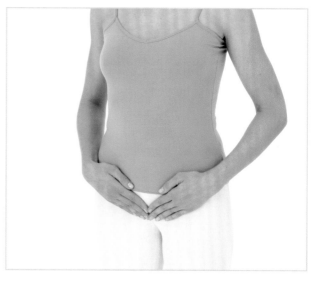

Front Position Three

Place your hands on either side of your navel, fingers touching in the middle. This position regulates sugar and fat metabolism (in the pancreas) and digestion, and helps ease powerful emotions such as fear, depression and frustration. It also helps to increase self-confidence.

Front Position Four

Place your hands over the pubic bone, in the shape of a V. For women, the fingertips should touch; for men the hands should rest further apart on the groin area. This treats the large intestine, bladder, urethra, sexual organs and menstrual disorders, and eases existential fears.

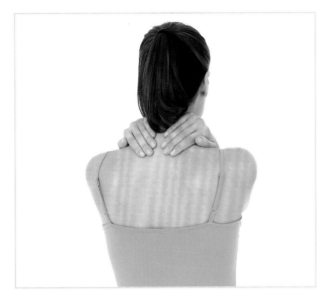

Back Position One

Place your hands on your upper shoulders, on either side of your spine. This position is helpful for relieving shoulder tension and back and neck problems, promotes relaxation, releases blocked emotions and helps difficulties with responsibility.

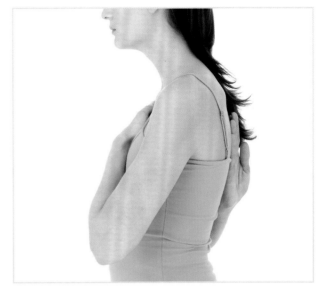

Back Position Two

Place one hand in the middle of your chest and the other at the same height on your back, palm facing out. This balances the thymus gland, harmonizes the heart, stimulates the immune system, increases enjoyment of life and confidence, and eases worries and depression. If you find it hard to reach between your shoulder blades, place your hands on your chest, one above the other.

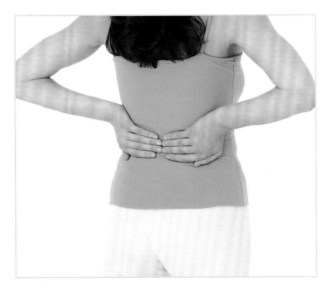

Back Position Three

Place your hands around your waist at kidney height, fingers pointing towards the spine. This position strengthens the kidneys, adrenal glands and nerves, promotes detoxification, eases stress and back pain, and reinforces self-esteem and confidence.

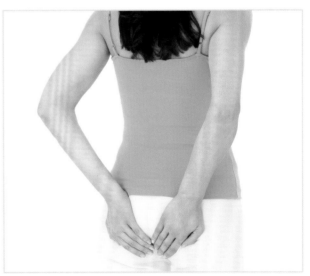

Back Position Four

Place your hands behind you so that your fingers are touching your coccyx, with your hands opening into a V. This position treats the sexual organs, digestion and the sciatic nerve, promotes creativity and confidence, and provides grounding.

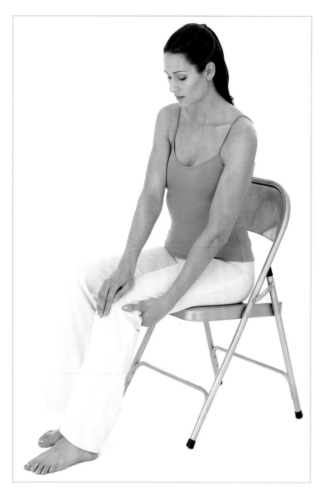

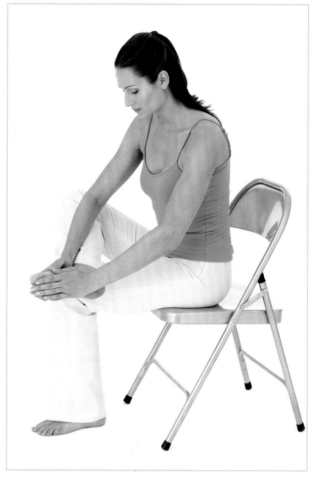

Knees

Place one hand on each knee. Alternatively, hold one hand underneath and one on top of the knee (in a 'sandwich') for 3–5 minutes, one knee at a time. This position is good for any knee problems, sport injuries or joint damage. Emotionally, it is connected with issues of fear and stepping forward in life.

Feet

Hold each foot with both hands, in a 'sandwich'. You are treating the foot reflex zones, which are located over the sole of each foot and correspond to all the organs in the body. This position also helps your own grounding and fortifies the first chakra.

Treating others

A full Reiki treatment for treating others is based on the following main hand positions. Placing your hands in these positions enables Reiki to flow into each chakra and in and around the physical and energy body. It is usual to start a Reiki treatment by first treating the head, then the front of the body, then the back of the body and finally the knees and feet.

Hands-off technique

Very rarely a receiver cannot bear to be touched. If this is the case, hold your hands above their body, treating and working in the aura, holding each hand position at a height that is comfortable for you. Maintain each position for 3–5 minutes, allowing an hour in total to complete the whole treatment.

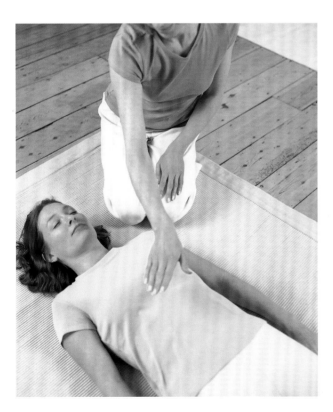

When working in the auric field, the Reiki energy will be absorbed by the physical body through the chakras in the same way as when being touched.

PRACTICAL TIPS

- It is important that both giver and receiver are comfortable during the treatment, and it is usually best for the receiver to lie down (use a massage table or cushioned mat). Tell the receiver that, if they need to, they can alter their position during treatment.
- Place your hands lightly, firmly and confidently, without exerting any pressure, in each new hand position. Lay your hands gently and adjust them to the receiver's body shape and contours; the better the contact between giver and receiver, the more the flow of Reiki energy is supported.
- Keep your fingers relaxed and together, your thumbs tucked into your hands.
- Most people like the touch of healing hands, finding it reassuring. Some receivers like to use a soft eye pillow to cover their eyes. Place this gently over the eyes after you have completed Head Position One. The soft pressure of the eye pillow soothes the eyeballs, which generally supports relaxation.

Trusting your intuition

While giving Reiki, trust your intuition. Sometimes you may sense that a particular area of the body needs more Reiki than elsewhere. Keep your hands there until the energy flow has normalized. During a treatment, you might feel strongly drawn to give Reiki to other places as well. Trust your judgement and place your hands wherever they are needed (see Treatment Guidelines, page 60).

The 17 basic hand positions

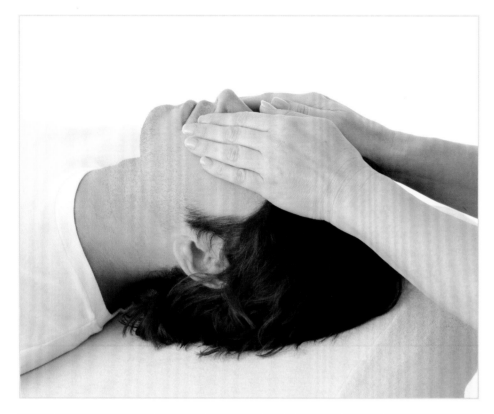

Head Position One

Lay your hands to the right and left of the nose, covering the forehead, eyes and cheeks. This position is good for treating the eyes and sinuses. It balances the pituitary and pineal glands. Use it for treating exhaustion, stress, colds, sinus disorders, eye disorders and allergies. Relaxing the eyes relaxes the whole body.

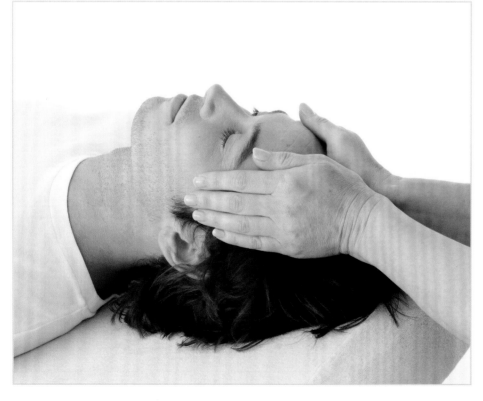

Head Position Two

Lay your hands on both sides of the head, above the ears, with the fingertips touching the temples, and the palms following the shape of the head. This position is good for treating the eye muscles and nerves. It balances the right and left sides of the brain and the body. It helps ease stress and excessive mental activity, calms the mind, helps learning and concentration difficulties, and also alleviates colds and headaches.

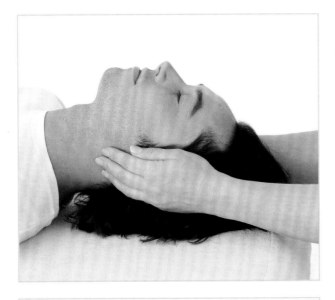

Head Position Three

Lay your hands over the ears. This position is good for treating the organs of balance and the pharynx. Use it to treat disturbances to the sense of balance, disorders of the outer and inner ear, noises or hissing in the ears, poor hearing and disorders of the nose and throat, as well as colds and flu.

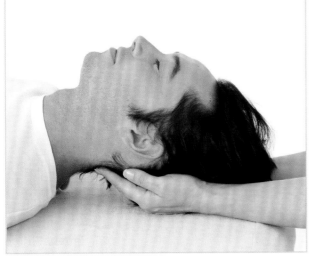

Head Position Four

Cup the back of the head with the fingertips over the medulla oblongata, an energy point where many nerves connect at the join between the head and neck. This position is good for treating the back of the head, eyes and nose, and helps to clarify thinking. Use it for calming powerful emotions such as fear, shock and tension, for headaches, eye disorders, colds, asthma, hay fever and digestive disorders.

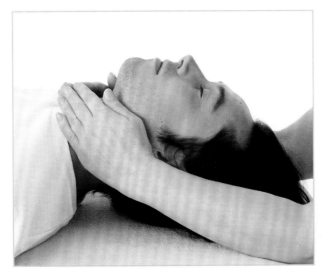

Head Position Five

Lay your hands at the sides and above the front part of the throat, but do not touch the throat directly. This position is good for treating the thyroid and parathyroid glands, larynx, vocal cords and lymph nodes. Use it for metabolic disorders, weight problems, heart palpitations and fibrillation, high or low blood pressure, sore throats, inflammation of the tonsils, flu, hoarseness and repressed or overacted aggressions. It promotes self-expression.

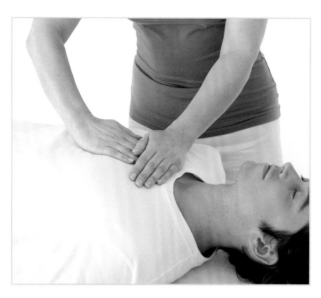

Front Position One

Lay one hand across the thymus gland, below the collarbone, the other at right angles to the first on the breastbone, in the middle of the chest (together the hands form a T). This position is good for treating the thymus gland, heart and lungs. It is related to the fourth chakra. Use it for fortifying the immune and lymphatic system, healing heart or lung disorders and for bronchitis, deafness, general weakness and depression.

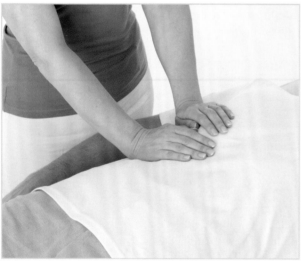

Front Position Two

Lay one hand on the lower ribs on the right side, below the chest, the other directly below it at waist level. This position is good for treating the liver and gallbladder, pancreas, duodenum and parts of the stomach and large intestine. Use it for liver and gallbladder disorders, such as hepatitis, gallstones, digestive disorders, metabolic disorders and detoxification problems. It also balances emotions such as anger and depression.

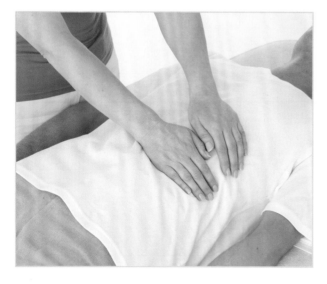

Front Position Three

Lay one hand on the lower ribs on the left side, below the chest, and the other directly below it at waist level. This position is good for treating the spleen, parts of the pancreas, large intestine, small intestine and stomach. Use it for disorders of the pancreas or spleen, diabetes, flu, infections, digestive disorders, anaemia and leukaemia. In AIDS and cancer, it helps to stabilize the immune system.

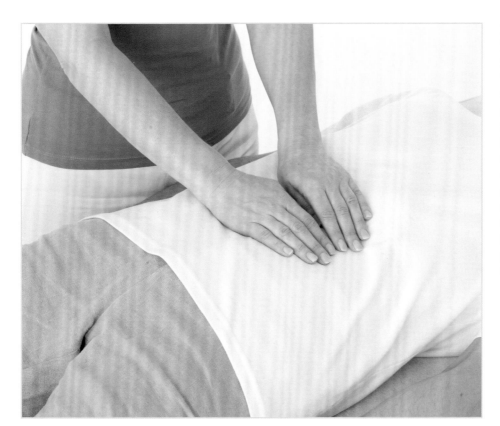

Front Position Four

Lay one hand above, and the other below, the navel. This position is good for treating the solar plexus, stomach, digestive organs, lymphatic system and intestines. It is related to the second and third chakras. Use it for stomach and intestinal disorders and for powerful emotions such as depression, fear and shock. It is also a good position for restoring energy and vitality.

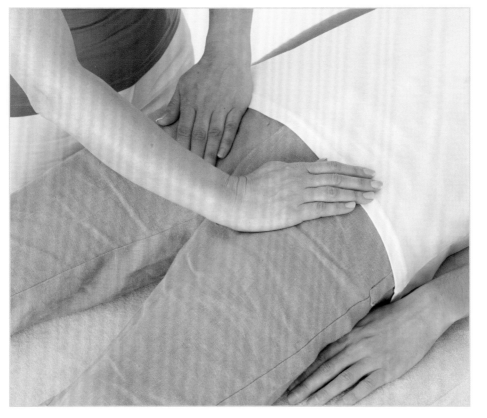

Front Position Five

This is also known as the V Position. For men, place your hands in the groin area, without touching the sexual organs. For women, lay both hands over the pubic bone. This position is good for treating the abdominal organs, intestines, bladder and urethra. It is related to the first chakra. Use it for urogenital, menstrual and menopausal disorders, appendix and digestive orders, cramps, back pain, ovarian tumours, uterus, bladder and prostate-gland problems.

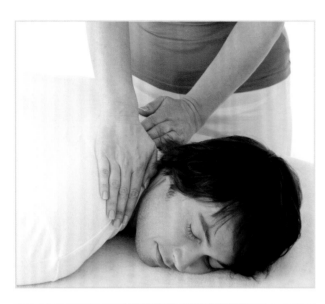

Back Position One

Lay both hands on the shoulders, with one hand to the left and the other to the right of the spine, hands facing in the same direction. This position is good for treating the nape of the neck and the shoulder muscles. Use it for easing tension in the shoulders and the nape of the neck, neck problems, stress, blocked emotions and problems with responsibility.

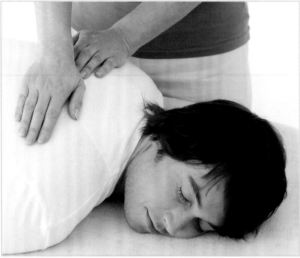

Back Position Two

Lay your hands on the shoulder blades, with the fingertips of one hand touching the base of the other palm. This position is good for treating shoulders, heart, lungs and upper back. Use it for lung and heart disorders, coughs, bronchitis, back and shoulder complaints, powerful emotional upsets and depression. It promotes the capacity for love, confidence and enjoyment.

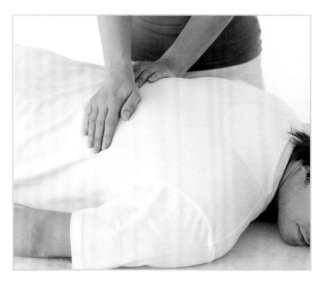

Back Position Three

Lay your hands on the lower ribs, above the kidneys. This position helps in the treatment of the adrenal glands, kidneys and nervous system. Use it for kidney disorders, allergies, detoxification, hay fever, shock from accidents, fears, stress and back pain. This releases the middle back and helps the receiver to let go of any stress and pain from the past.

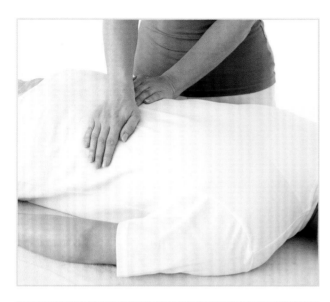

Back Position Four

If the receiver has a long back, lay your hands on the lower part of the back at hip level. This position helps sciatica and lower back pain, strengthens the lymph and nerves, supports creativity and sexuality, and also eases hip problems.

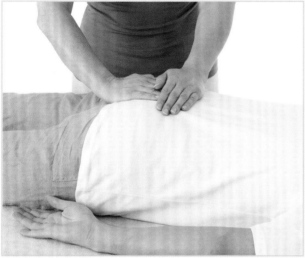

Back Position Five (A) – T Position

Lay one hand across the sacrum, the other at right angles to the first, over the coccyx to form a T. This position is good for treating the intestines, the urogenital system and the sciatic nerve. It is related to the first chakra and helps existential fears. Use it for haemorrhoids, digestive complaints, intestinal inflammations, bladder disorders, the prostate gland, vaginal disorders and sciatic pain.

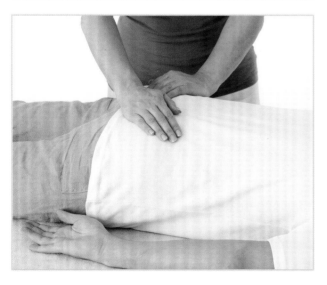

Back Position Five (B) – V Position

Alternatively, place your hands in a V shape on the receiver's buttocks, with the fingertips of one hand (the point of the V) directly on the coccyx. This position encourages energy to flow more freely up the spine, which results in harmonizing the nervous system and promoting confidence.

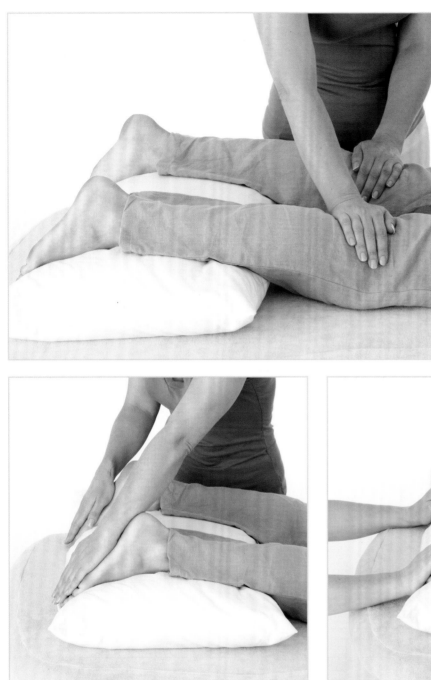

Knee Hollow Position

Cover the hollows of the knees with your hands. This position is good for treating all parts of the knee joint. Use it for joint damage, sports injuries and blocks that interrupt the energy flow from the feet to the lower back. This position also deals emotionally with the issue of fear, especially the fear of dying.

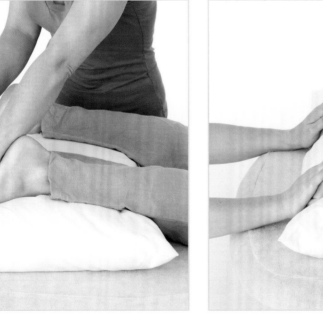

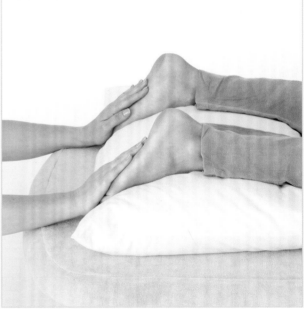

Sole Positions (A or B)

Lay your hands on the soles of the feet, with the fingertips covering the toes (A). In this position, the receiver may experience a release of energy. If you point your fingertips towards the heels (B), the receiver will sense a strong energy flow from the feet to the head.

The Sole Positions are good for treating the foot reflex zones for all organs, which are located over the entire sole of the foot. Use them for fortification of the first chakra and for the grounding of all the chakras and regions of the body.

16 additional hand positions

The additional hand positions are useful when the receiver is experiencing physical or emotional problems and you want to give extra Reiki to those specific areas.

Suitable purposes

Appropriate conditions include sciatic pain, neck problems, poor leg circulation, fears and tension, hip-joint pain, stress symptoms, headaches, multiple sclerosis, back problems, metabolism and weight problems. Hold your hands in position for 3–5 minutes. If you experience noticeable sensations of heat, cold, tingling, shaking or a 'drawing in' of the energy in a particular hand position, hold that position for a while longer, until the sensation beneath your hands feels 'normal' again.

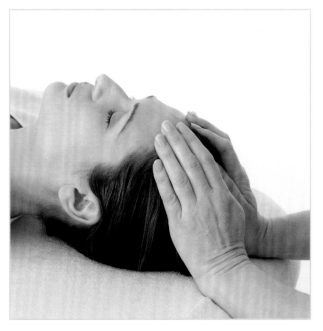

Head position
Lay both hands on the cap of the skull. This position is good for treating cerebral fissures and the capillary system. Use it for stress, headaches, balancing disorders and for centring. For multiple sclerosis, give regular and intensive treatment.

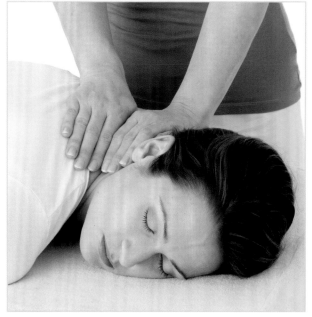

Neck-vertebra position
Lay one hand on the nape of the neck and the other on the top neck vertebra. Use this position for treating whiplash injury, pain in the bones, heart, spine and nerve and neck problems.

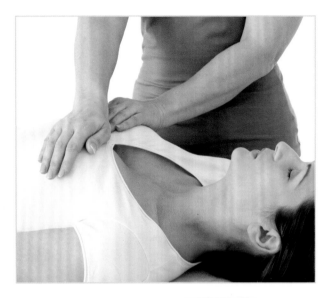

Breast and chest position

Lay the hands on both sides of the chest. This position helps to harmonize the male and female sides. Ask the receiver beforehand if they feel comfortable being touched here.

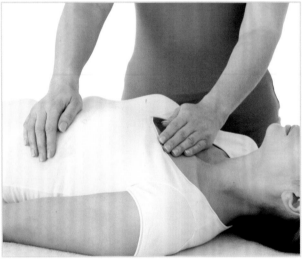

Spleen and thymus-gland position

Lay your left hand on the lower left side of the ribcage (spleen area) and place your right hand below the collarbone, across the thymus gland. This position is good for treating the lymphatic system and the spleen, helping with problems of the immune system and auto-immune disorders.

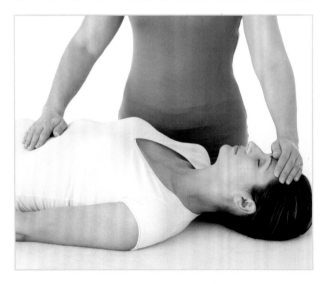

Head and belly position

Lay one hand on the forehead and the other on the belly (just below the navel). This position has a calming and centring effect, and promotes spiritual equilibrium and general well-being.

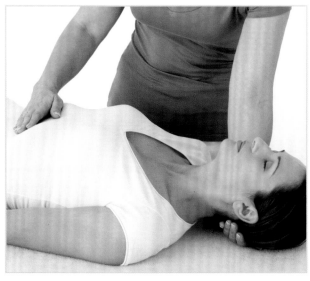

Head and solar-plexus position

Lay one hand on the back of the head and the other on the solar plexus. This position calms the nervous system and relaxes those suffering from stress and shock.

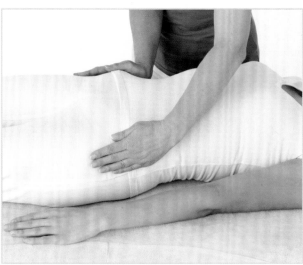

Hip-joints position

Lay the hands on the left and right hips. This position is good for treating the hip joints, varicose veins, leg pain and the gall point of the meridian system.

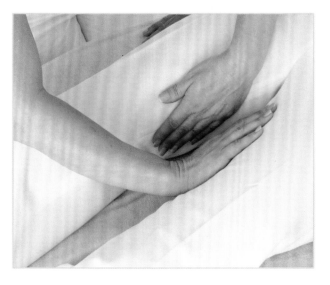

Inner-thighs position

Lay one hand flat on the inside of each thigh (fingertips pointing in opposite directions). This position is effective for treating the intestines. Emotions and tensions are also released; this is a let-go position for deep-seated fears.

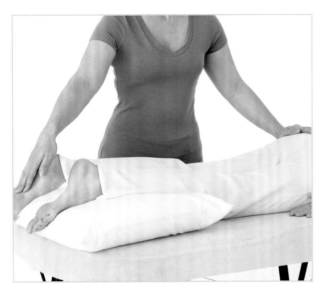

Buttocks, legs and heels position

Lay one hand directly on one buttock or over the sacrum, and the other on the heel on the same side. Whenever possible, treat both sides. This position is good for treating sciatic pain. Treat the whole leg, from buttocks to heels, by placing your hands on the back side of the whole leg, starting with the upper legs/thighs, moving down to the knees, calves and ankles, and finishing off with the soles of the feet.

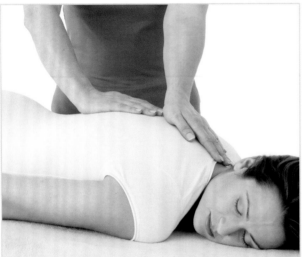

Spine position

Lay your hands, one after the other, first on the upper part of the spine, then on the lower part. Give treatment as far as the coccyx, and end with Back Position Five (A) or (B) (see page 139). The spine position is helpful for back problems, disc wear and degenerative diseases.

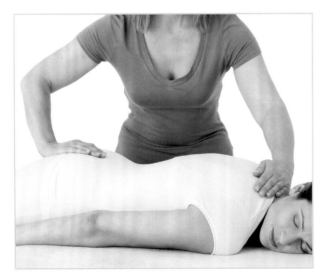

Coccyx and top of neck

Place one hand covering the coccyx and the other hand on top of the neck. Keep both hands in this position until the flow of energy feels the same in both hands. You are treating the spine and in particular the seventh vertebra. This position balances the energy of the whole spine. You can also try it on someone who is suffering from a hangover, as it is supposed to counteract the negative side-effects of alcohol.

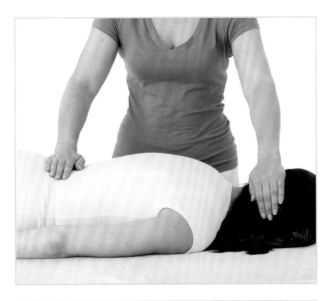

Lower back and back of head

Lay one hand on the lower back and the other on the back of the head. This position is suitable for ending your treatment, as it deeply relaxes and calms the nervous system. It supports a feeling of safety and security.

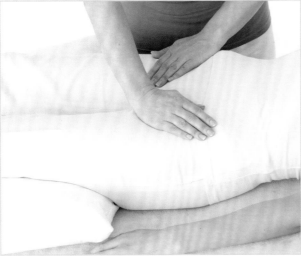

Groin area

Lay both hands on the front of the body in the groin area. Giving Reiki here is good for the circulation in the legs, for low blood pressure and the lymphatic system. This position also strengthens the energy of the first chakra (the will to live and issues of security), supports fertility and improves the immune system.

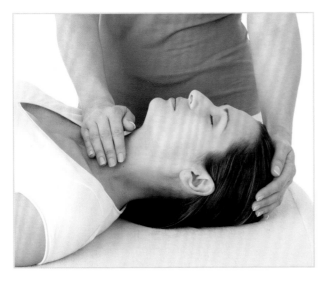

Throat and top of head

Place one hand on the front of the throat (fifth chakra) and lay the other hand on the centre of the top of the head (seventh chakra). This position is beneficial for the thyroid, pineal and pituitary glands, as well as the hypothalamus. It balances the metabolism, and is useful when you are experiencing weight problems (over- or underweight) and for older people whose metabolism has started to slow down. It is also beneficial for women going through the menopause, as it affects the hypothalamus, which controls the release of hormones in the body.

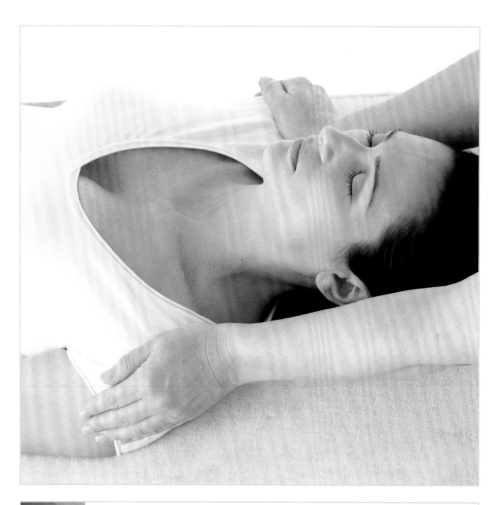

Shoulders, arms and hands

Place one hand on top of each shoulder where the shoulder curves, touching the shoulders and upper arms, fingertips pointing downwards towards the arms and hands. This position helps to release tension in the shoulders. After 2 or 3 minutes, start treating each arm separately by placing one hand on top of the right arm in the shoulder area and the other hand on the right elbow and then on the wrist. At the end, touch the whole palm of the hand. This position allows healing energy to run through the arms and hands. Treat until you feel that the energy is balanced. Then treat the left arm in the same way.

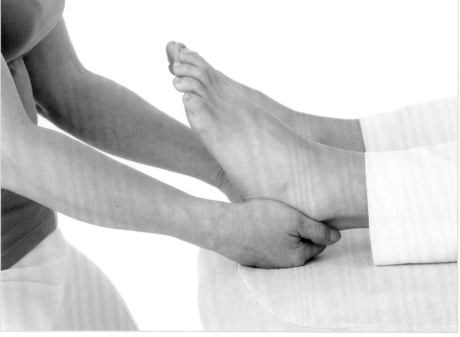

Feet, ankles, heels and toes

The feet have energy zones, called foot reflex zones, which correspond to all parts of the body. Giving Reiki to the soles of the feet, the ankles, heels, toes and top of the feet sends the healing energy to every organ and to other related points in the physical body.

Short Reiki treatment

If there is no time for a full Reiki treatment, then a form of short treatment is very useful. You can use it when someone needs to 'recharge their batteries', for example when travelling, or in any other stressful situation, such as experiencing a headache or tension. An additional bonus is that all the chakras are balanced at the same time. The short treatment is given in a sitting position, on a chair.

Smoothing the aura

Start your treatment by smoothing the aura from head to foot (see page 62), in a downward movement. This has a calming effect.

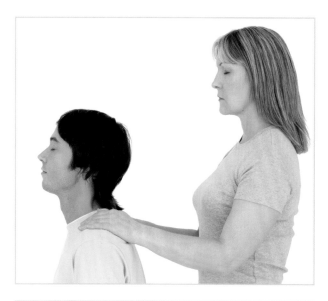

Position One

Lay your hands on the middle of each shoulder. This treats tension in the shoulders, arms and lower back, and helps treat shock.

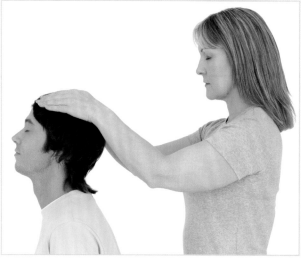

Position Two

Lay your hands on the top of the head, with the seventh chakra free (leaving a little gap between your hands). This harmonizes and supports the function of the brain and is helpful for relieving pressure in the head, dizziness, indigestion and stomach cramps.

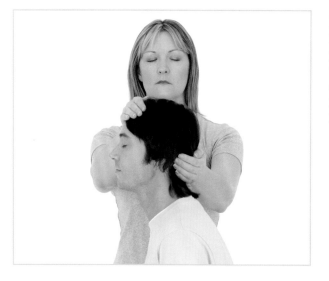

Position Three

Lay one hand on the place where the back of the head joins the spine (over the medulla oblongata), the other in the middle of the forehead. This position harmonizes the energy between the sixth chakra and the back of the head, and affects the pituitary and pineal glands. It is helpful for headaches, nosebleeds, colds and flu.

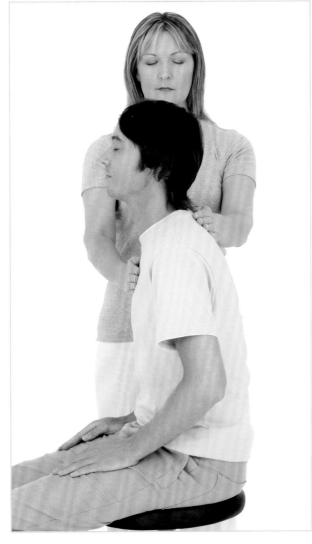

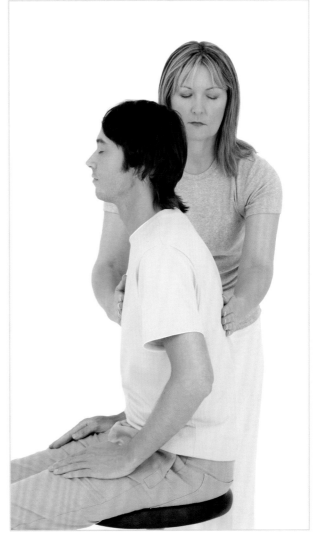

Position Four

Lay one hand on the thymus gland below the collarbone and the other at the same height on the upper back, below the seventh neck vertebra. This position treats the immune system, lungs, lower back, headaches, colds, coughs, premenstrual problems and bone complaints.

Position Five

Lay one hand on the heart chakra and the other in the opposite position on the back, one hand-width lower, covering the adrenals. This treats the heart, adrenals, gallbladder and pancreas, and helps with allergies, asthma, coughs, sleeplessness, nervousness and fears.

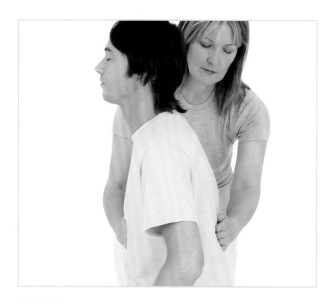

Position Six

Lay one hand on the stomach, covering the third chakra (solar-plexus area), and the other at the same height on the back, above waist level, in the kidney area. This treats the adrenals, kidneys, sciatic nerve, pancreas and spleen. It has a calming effect and helps with flatulence, nausea and oedema or water retention.

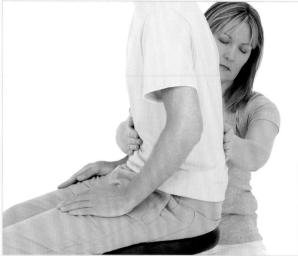

Position Seven

Lay one hand covering the navel and the other at the same height on the back, above the sacrum. This treats constipation, tachycardia, insulin levels, incontinence, oedema and shock. It advances digestion and the absorption of nutrition, and increases energy.

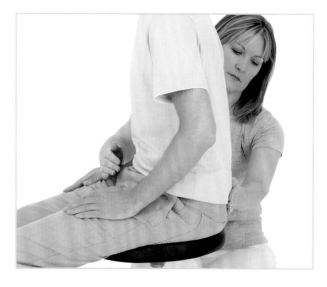

Position Eight

Lay one hand on the lower abdomen above the pubic bone and the other directly opposite on the lower back, on the coccyx. In this position you might want to keep your hands a few inches over the physical body and treat through the receiver's aura. This has the same effect as when touching, because the energy permeates the physical body. This position treats the lymphatic system, prostate gland, bladder and reproductive organs. It helps with constipation, sleeplessness and menstrual pains, and supports blood circulation.

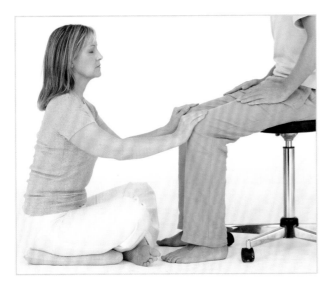

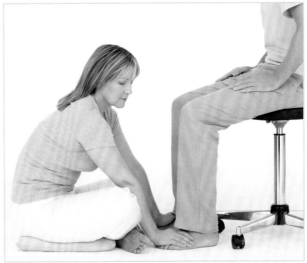

Knees and feet

If you have time, treat the knees and feet as shown, holding them in a 'sandwich' between the hands, one at a time. The knee position is useful for joint damage and sports injuries, and when energy blockages interrupt the flow from torso to feet. Treating the feet gives a good grounding for all the chakras and regions of the body, and in particular fortifies the first chakra. The receiver will sense a strengthened energy flow from feet to head.

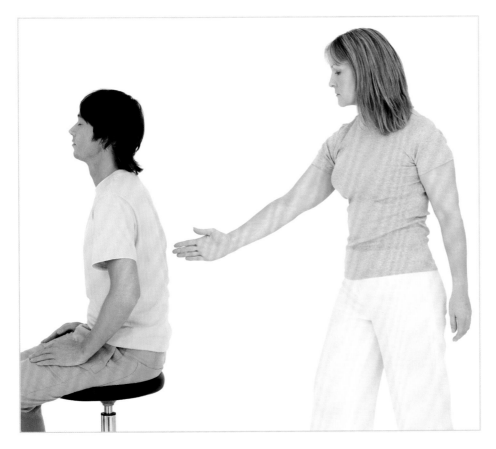

Spine

End the treatment by stroking upwards from the sacral region, directing the fingertips of one hand along the vertebrae of the spine in an upward movement. This refreshes energy and strengthens the body.

Group Reiki

In group treatment, we share Reiki energy with other Reiki practitioners and friends. Reiki is a means of non-verbal communication that creates intimacy between giver and receiver. We tune into the other person and sense where our hands are needed. Sharing Reiki is like sharing quality time with each other and enriches relationships. Group treatments are especially effective if anyone has a severe illness, since the Reiki power flows more intensely and many hand positions are covered at the same time.

Group work of three or more

The receiver lies down and receives Reiki from the rest of the group members. The number can range from 3–7 people. The treatment time is usually shorter (about 20 minutes for each treatment) than for a normal treatment. Take it in turns, so that each person gives and receives. Each giver can choose to treat a different area. There should be no talking during treatment time.

Instructions

1 One of the givers smoothes the aura, stroking with both hands from the top of the head down over the feet. Repeat this three times. It helps the receiver to relax.

2 Now all the givers treat the front of the body for about 10 minutes. Use specific hand positions or work intuitively. One person can treat the head, while two others place their hands on either side of the torso and another works on the legs and feet. Then ask the receiver to turn over and treat the back in a similar way, for another 10 minutes.

3 At the end of the treatment, one giver smoothes the aura (twice downwards and the last stroke upwards, to strengthen the energy).

Reiki sandwich

This treatment is performed in a group of three, and lasts for 15 minutes. The receiver should sit in the middle and is treated simultaneously by two givers, one sitting behind and the other in front.

Instructions

1 First, one of the givers smoothes the aura, as in Step 1 on the left.

2 Then the givers place their hands at the same time, intuitively, on different areas of the receiver's body. The treatment can be done from the front, back and the sides.

3 Finally, smooth the aura again and swap places, so that the roles are changed and each person takes turns giving and receiving.

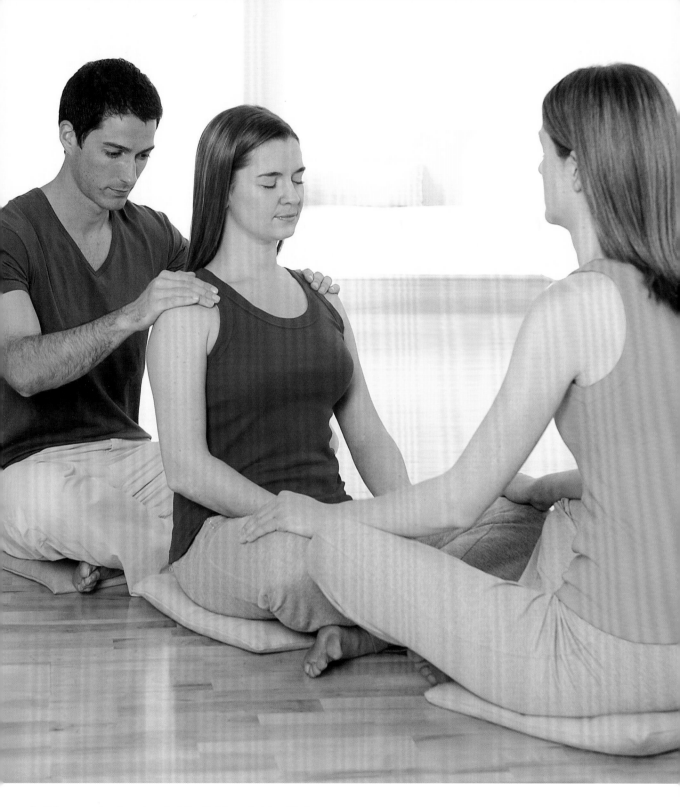

In this group treatment, called the Reiki sandwich, with the receiver sitting between two givers, the hands of the latter can be placed anywhere on the body.

Reiki energy circle

The energy circle is ideal for meetings and seminars. You can use it at work (at the beginning or end of meetings) to create better communication with colleagues and help everyone feel more present. Each individual feels a part of the circle, connected with the larger whole. Hold hands for 5–10 minutes.

Instructions

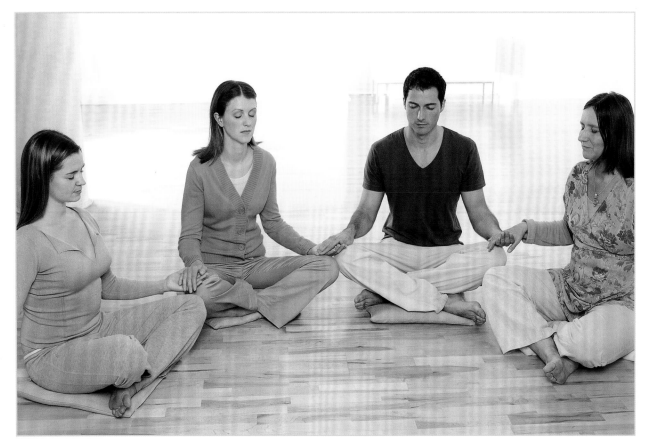

1 Stand or sit in a circle, each person taking a few deep breaths and relaxing the shoulders.

2 Hold hands with the people on either side, so that your right palm faces down, giving to the person on your right side. Your left palm faces up, receiving from the person on your left. Make sure your arms are held comfortably.

3 Receive the energy from your left (female) side, letting it pass though your palm, then along your left arm into the chest area (fourth chakra), before flowing down your right arm (male side) and out through the right palm, into the hand of the person sitting on your right.

4 Notice any sensations in your hands and body while giving and receiving at the same time. Become aware of the connection to everyone in the circle.

Reiki hug

The Reiki hug is a very effective and nourishing way to exchange loving energy. It is also a good way to thank someone else for giving you a treatment, or simply to connect on a deeper level, exchanging energy from heart to heart.

Instructions

1 When hugging, connect the upper bodies so that the left side of your chest is touching the left side of the other person's chest. In this way, the energy can flow more freely. Your hands can rest on the other person's upper or lower back. Make sure you are both comfortable.

2 Stay as long you like in this relaxing, loving embrace. If you can let a feeling of melting occur, that is wonderful and will make you feel that you are becoming one with the other person.

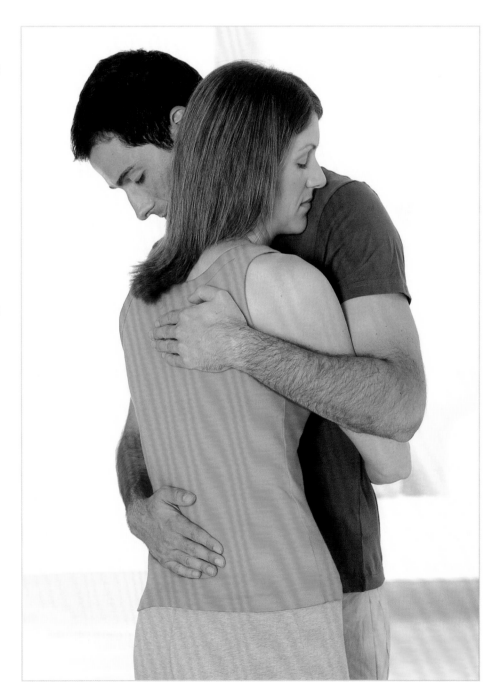

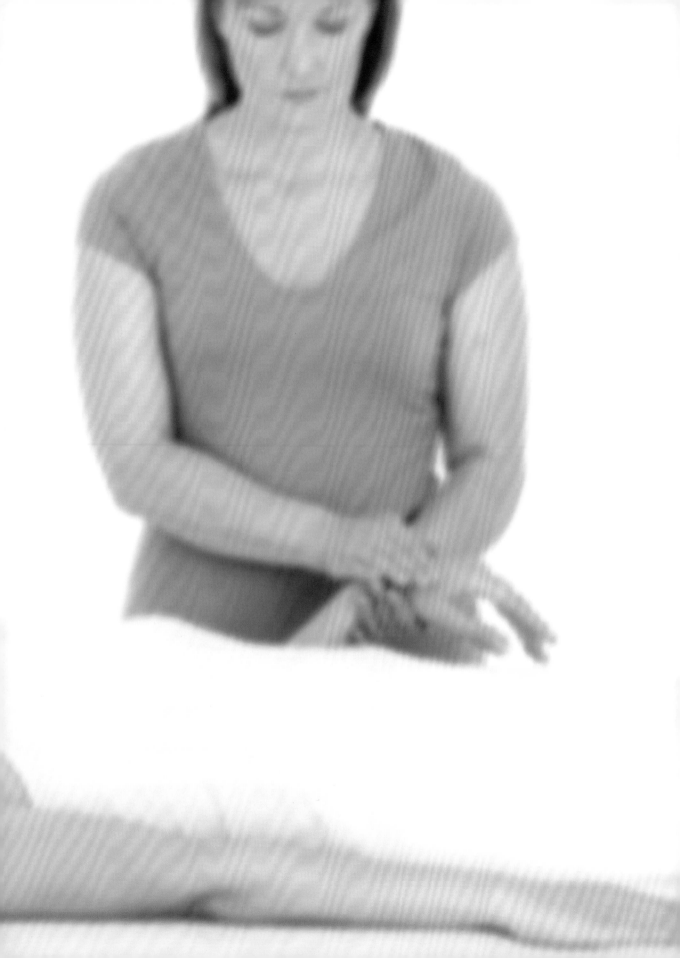

Reiki for common ailments

Our natural state as human beings is to be healthy and happy. However, an important challenge in life is to deal with its many different facets – some of them negative. This training is a process of growing into the mysteries and depths of the healing process, requiring dedication, sincerity and experience. The student may be motivated to find out more about the Self and to use this wisdom to help others discover themselves and to love and heal themselves.

Finding the real reason for illness

Reiki enables us to get in touch with the cause of disease or bodily imbalance, because it works on the levels of body, mind, emotions and spirit. Both giver and receiver need to listen carefully to any messages from the body and mind, because these can be subtle.

The body–mind connection

When receiving Reiki, the healing energy supports the body's natural ability to heal itself as a priority. This means that the energy releases negativity, blockages and toxins from the body. If we wish, we can speed up this healing process by looking for the reason behind the physical problem, with the intention of finding, healing and eliminating its true cause. This involves a commitment to examine the problem honestly. The main condition for healing is the receiver's willingness to be open to change, shifts of attitudes, behaviour and outlook. Without change there can be no spiritual growth, and this is required for healing to come about.

There is a constant interaction between body, psyche and emotions; positive energy (joy, love) keeps the body flexible and pliant, while suppressed energy (anger, sadness) and unfulfilled desires (frustration, disappointment) create blockages, initially in the energy body and later in the physical body. If these are not listened to, they can create imbalance and disease in the body in later life. Other factors, such as genes, environment and pollution, nutrition and physical activity, also influence the body's state of health.

Tools

The mind is a powerful tool that can work for and against our well-being and health. Illness is a result of imbalance, often caused by an unconscious mental attitude and belief, which are based on emotional reactions to events in our lives. This chapter can help you to gain insights into yourself and others to help determine what the emotional causes of your problems could be.

Start by asking yourself the following questions:
'What are my fears?'
'What am I thinking?'
'What am I holding back and not expressing?'
'How is this manifesting physically in me at this moment in time?

Listen to your body and heart; you will find the answers within you.

The Mental Healing technique learnt in the Second Degree (see page 86) also gives you valuable tools to look for the reason beneath disease or for emotional problems about the past or present. In this chapter you will learn about possible causes for illness and interactions between body, mind and soul, as well as ways in which you can use Reiki to heal them.

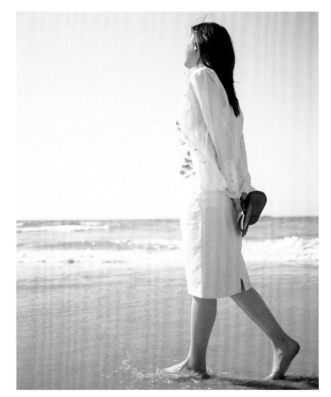

A sense of peace and calm results from the harmonious flow of energy between body, mind and spirit. Reiki helps to promote this by supporting your natural well-being.

Possible causes of illness and disease

Eyes: Inner seeing, feeling and hearing (third eye), not being seen by others, not wanting to see what is going on; connected to the sinus passages, where stored tears are held.

Teeth: Feelings of indecisiveness over a long time.

Throat: Swallowed anger, hurt and other feelings, inability to express yourself; throat blockages caused by choking on words, thoughts or beliefs, not saying what needs to be said, inability to tell the truth.

Upper back: Right side – stored anger, giving too much, holding on to irritation, striking out or back, holding out or back, defending yourself through an imbalance between giving and receiving; left side – stored sadness, grief, sorrow, loss, guilt.

Arms and hands: Issues of giving (right hand) and receiving (left hand) love, fear of letting go, holding on to things and people (what issues in life can you not cope with?).

Tailbone: Survival, fear of success, fear of aliveness and action, kundalini activity.

Knees: Inflexibility in thinking, obstinacy, indecision (what decision are you afraid to make?).

Ankles: Understanding related to thinking; fear of death and dying (what changes do you need to make in your life?).

Right side of the body: Represents the masculine, extrovert energies of survival (money and job issues), adventurousness, outgoing activity, aggressiveness, logical thinking and exertion of the will.

Nose: Sense and smell, sexual response; a cry for love and the need for self-recognition.

Ears: Blocking out what you do not want to hear, not being heard by others, unwilling to listen to inner guidance; related to high blood pressure, balance and clarity.

Mouth: Survival, how we deal with security, the capacity to take in new ideas.

Neck and shoulders: Carrying burdens and responsibilities for family, business, the world and others; feelings of guilt and stress.

Chest/heart/lungs: Relationship issues, heartbreak, loss, fear, sadness, rejection, hurt, feelings of worthlessness, suppressed emotions, low self-esteem, feeling controlled by others; holding back out of fear of being alive, low energy, coughing up pain, blockages of love and imbalances between giving and receiving.

Lower back: Stored anger and resentment, feeling unsupported, trying to be perfect, money issues and indefinable fears, sexual imbalance, barriers against the opposite sex and issues with sexual abuse.

Legs: Associated with progress in life, fear of the future and of change, family issues (what is holding you back in life?).

Feet: Represents what you stand for and your grounding in life, standing up for yourself and others; associated with security and survival, reaching goals and fear of taking the next step in life.

Left side of the body: Represents the feminine energies of nourishment, receptivity, creativity, intuition and gentle and loving energies.

List of organs related to behaviour and illness

Thyroid: Feelings of being humiliated and emotional charges of accusation.

Lungs: Losing the ability to receive and breathing problems mean that you refuse to take life in; pneumonia means that you are tired of life and will not let yourself heal.

Liver: Indications of anger and fear stored over long periods of time.

Stomach: Fear and dread that you do not have the ability to assimilate the new and unknown; things are swallowed and are difficult to digest, such as old learned patterns and conditioning from family, peers and teachers; an ulcer is anger eating away at the gut; anxious feelings create a nervous stomach; fear of disapproval causes indigestion of old thoughts, feelings and ideas that do not fit into your life any more.

Gallbladder: Indications of anger turned into bitterness; hard feelings and development of condemning pride.

Intestinal tract: Constipation indicates holding feelings in, usually anger, fear and guilt; feelings of being stuck in the past, refusal to move on to new ideas. Diarrhoea and colitis indicate letting go of old feelings, thoughts and ideas without actually dealing with them; fear and rejection of things that may nourish you.

Genitals: Survival issues, fear of life, relating to the first chakra.

Prostate: Sexual guilt, anger against women; feelings of powerlessness, helplessness and issues with birth, incest and sexual abuse.

Testicles: Represent masculine energy; problems in this area can result from a fear and rejection of male energy.

Heart: Indications that you may be lacking joy with an inability to love yourself and others; the heart is the centre for love and security.

Spleen: Being obsessed with things; storage of unfinished business with past relationships; could relate to the death of a loved one (parent or partner) or to a job or lifestyle that creates unwelcome connections with the past.

Adrenals and kidneys: Overactivity of the sympathetic nervous system, adrenal rushes, healing of the entire auto-immune system. Issues: self-criticism, feelings of shame and disappointment in life and in yourself; being confused; indications of unexpressed feeling, particularly anger; treat for shock, trauma, illness, surgery, emotional imbalance, stress, allergies, low energy and fear response.

Pancreas: The sweetness has gone from life; the spark, spice and zest are absent, characterized by being too nice or 'sugary'.

Abdomen: The seat of the emotions, containing the deepest feelings, centre of sexuality, digestive system.

Ovaries/uterus: Indicates stored anger against men; unresolved issues with birth, abortion, miscarriage, rape, incest, abuse, fear, guilt and anger about sexuality.

Bladder: Holding on to old feelings, such as stored anger; this can be related to fear and guilt around sexuality; fear of letting go accompanied by anxiety.

Reiki in first aid

Reiki can be applied directly as first aid. It has a very calming effect on the nervous system, particularly when people are in shock after an accident.

Supporting stress

In an emergency the body automatically goes into 'fight or flight' mode, whereby the adrenal cortex increases adrenaline production, which supports our reaction to extreme stress. The adrenaline is transported in the blood to the body's cells, making the person ready for action and reaction. However, the adrenal glands are soon exhausted and are then under tension and stress. You can help people in emergency situations by calming and balancing them with Reiki.

Burns

Give Reiki just above, but not touching, the actual injury for 20–30 minutes, possibly at intervals. The pain may initially worsen, before beginning to subside. If you can give Reiki straight away, blisters are less likely to form.

Wounds

Give Reiki just above the wound (holding your hands over the body, without touching it). Later, after medical attention when the dressing has been applied, give Reiki through the bandage.

Heart attack

Call for emergency medical help immediately. In the meantime, give Reiki to the upper and lower belly, but not directly to the heart.

Fear

Lay your hands on the the chakra (solar-plexus area), adrenal glands (in the middle back) and the back of the head (over the medulla oblongata). Alternatively, carry out Mental Healing (see page 86) and Distant Healing (see page 96).

Insect bites

Give Reiki directly on the site of the bite for 20–30 minutes. If you can do this immediately, you may be able to minimize the swelling.

Bruising and sprains

Give Reiki immediately, directly on the site of the bruise or sprain, for 20–30 minutes.

Broken bones

After the bone has been set by a health professional, lay your hands gently on the plaster. The pain might increase a little at the outset as the healing begins.

Shock

Call emergency help immediately. In the meantime, give Reiki to the solar plexus (third chakra) and the adrenal glands simultaneously. Alternatively, treat the back of the head and the adrenal glands together. Later on, treat the shoulders or just hold the injured person's hand; place your hands wherever you can comfortably reach.

'One morning our kitchen toaster started burning. My son was terribly shocked, because of the fire. I placed my hands on his body, on the middle front side and opposite on the back and he immediately calmed down.'

Brigitte

Warning: Reiki is not a substitute for emergency medical attention and should only be used to calm and comfort before medical assistance arrives.

Treating specific ailments

When treating specific ailments, we first need to determine whether they are acute or chronic. An acute ailment is recent and responds rapidly and directly to Reiki energy, while chronic problems need intense, prolonged treatment.

Acute ailments

When a receiver with acute symptoms is treated, the Reiki power is absorbed immediately and in large amounts, which can result in bringing out the symptoms of the health problem more strongly. These self-healing reactions are part of the healing and are called a 'healing crisis'. As in homeopathy, a climax is reached so that the

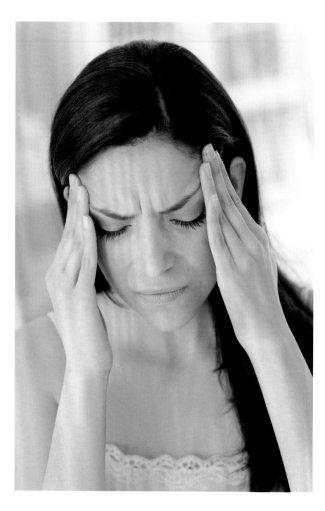

toxic energy can leave the body. Self-healing reactions are a good sign and indicate that healing is taking place. They usually subside within a few hours or days. The receiver is generally free of symptoms after the third day following the Reiki treatment.

Chronic ailments

Chronic complaints require intense treatment for several hours, over a prolonged period. Here the healing crisis, with its self-healing reactions, takes place in a later part of the healing process. At this point the receiver might experience a relapse, when the Reiki energy and the toxins react against each other, before the Reiki energy can clear the body of toxins. When a healing crisis is taking place, it resembles a chronic illness becoming acute again. At this point it is vital to continue Reiki treatments, since you have arrived at the core of the disease and the remaining toxins are being released. However, a healing crisis is not always apparent when treating chronic diseases. Sometimes physical symptoms may subside gently, without coming to a climax.

Practicalities

The recommended time for remaining in each hand position during the treatment is 3–5 minutes, but you may hold the position longer, especially when you sense that the receiver is absorbing a lot of Reiki energy. Sometimes you might stay in one position for 10 or 15 minutes.

All treatment positions given here are described for treating someone else, but you can also use them on yourself, as self-treatment. You might need to adjust the hand position to be able to reach the same areas of the body – simply use your common sense when making adjustments in this way.

A receiver suffering from an acute ailment may experience symptoms to a greater degree after a Reiki treatment, but this self-healing reaction is a sign that healing is happening.

Headache

Headaches can be caused by a cold or flu, excessive tension created by worry, not drinking enough water, toxins being unable to be released from the body and other reasons.

Recommended: Drink plenty of water and perhaps use the Bach Flower Rescue Remedy.

Treatment

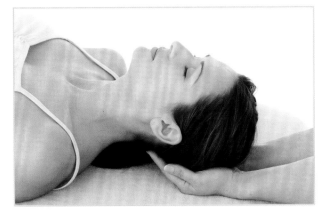

1 Lay both your hands directly on the area of pain that requires treatment.

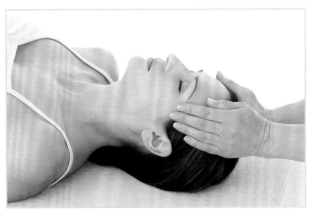

2 Place your hands on both sides of the head above the ears, fingertips touching the temples and palms, following the curve of the head, in Head Position Two.

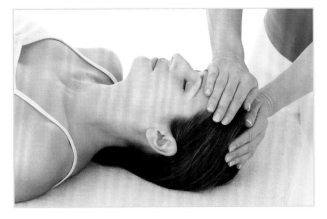

3 Hold the back of the head with the fingertips over the medulla oblongata, in Head Position Four. This releases tension as well as pain.

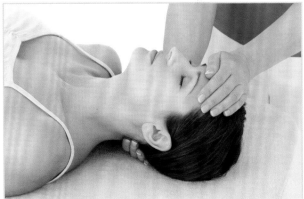

4 Lay one hand on the back of the head (slide your hand underneath) over the medulla oblongata; place the other hand over the forehead (sixth chakra). This reduces stress and facilitates meditation; it is also good for multiple sclerosis, epilepsy and insomnia.

Migraine

Migraine is a severe form of headache. Common migraines may develop into a throbbing pain on one or both sides of the head, whereas a classic migraine often begins with visual disturbance that subsides to be followed by a one-sided headache. Migraines tend to be recurrent and may be caused by stress, food sensitivity, bright lights, loud noises and menstruation. They are often accompanied by nausea, vomiting and stomach complaints, and indicate an imbalance between liver, gallbladder and spleen.

Recommended: Drink lots of water and perhaps use the Bach Flower Rescue Remedy.

Treatment

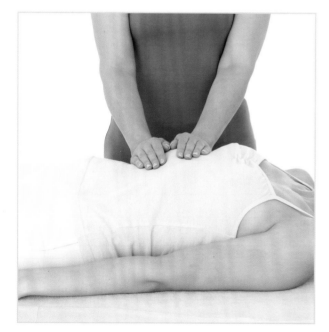

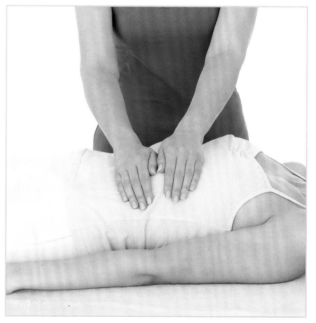

1 Lay both hands next to each other over the lower ribcage on the right side of the body, in Front Position Two.

2 Move both hands opposite over the lower ribs and waist on the left side of the body, in Front Position Three. These positions treat the liver and gallbladder, and support the spleen and digestion.

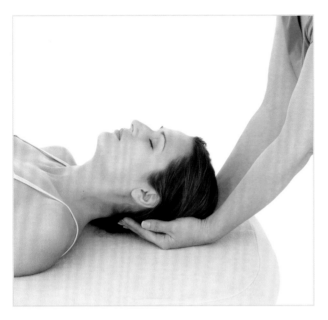

3 Now place your hands on the back of the head, with the fingertips over the medulla oblongata, in Head Position Four. This position releases tension in the head and helps digestive disorders.

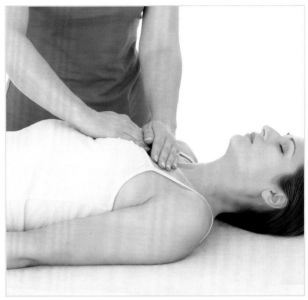

4 Place one hand horizontally across the thymus gland and the other at right angles to the first, in the middle of the chest, in Front Position One. This gives you strength and supports the immune system.

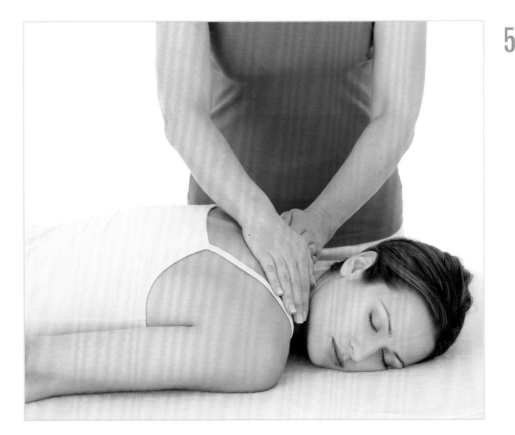

5 Place your hands on the upper shoulders, one hand to the left and the other to the right of the spine (with the middle fingers of one hand touching the channel of the spine), in Back Position One. This position is good for releasing tension in the neck and shoulders, for stress and blocked emotions. Additionally, you can use some of the positions for treating a headache (see page 163).

Neck, shoulder and upper-back pain

Tension in the neck, shoulder muscles and upper back is often caused by stress, poor posture, lack of exercise or an imbalance in the liver and gallbladder. Pain can also be caused by inflammation in the shoulder joints, whiplash injury, or 'sore bones' and growing pains. Emotional causes for pain in the upper back, shoulders and neck can include holding back emotions or feeling overloaded with responsibility. All the following positions release tension and pain in the neck, shoulders and upper back.

Recommended: Find out the source of the back pain. Use daily stretching exercises (morning is best) to loosen and tone the related muscles. Take regular aerobic exercise and brisk walks. Reduce stress levels and repressed emotions such as anger and fear. Therapeutic massage and chiropractic treatment can be beneficial.

CASE STUDY **LOWER-BACK PAIN**

CLIENT PROFILE
Eleanor (a Second Degree Reiki Trainee) had arranged with her grown-up nephew Roy to send him some healing on his lower back, where he had been having problems.

THE REIKI TREATMENT
She went through the sequence (Back Position One to Five), and when she put her hands on his shoulders (Back Position One), it felt as though they were moving backwards and forwards, almost like a kneading action. When she moved her hands closer to the spine, the feeling came back. Once she'd finished the treatment, she asked Roy if he'd had a problem with his shoulders – he said he had; they'd been very sore and had a deep ache in them. Eleanor asked him how they were and he was rather surprised to say they were better – the pain had gone.

Treatment

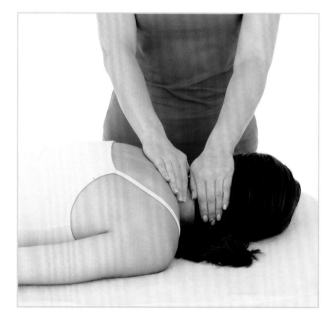

1 Place one hand on the nape of the neck and the other on the top neck vertebra.

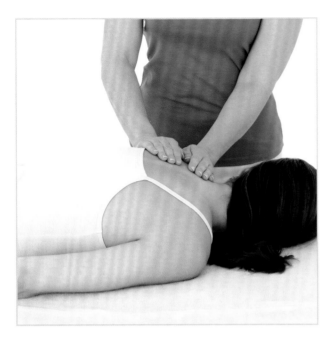

2 Place your palms next to each other on the left shoulder, with the base of the palms on the shoulder muscle, fingers pointing towards the spine.

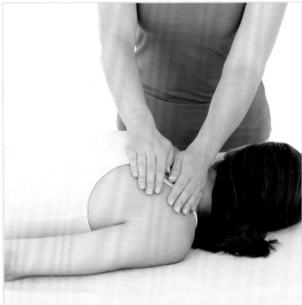

3 Move your hands onto the right upper shoulder, this time with the base of the palms on the spine and the fingers pointing to the shoulder muscle.

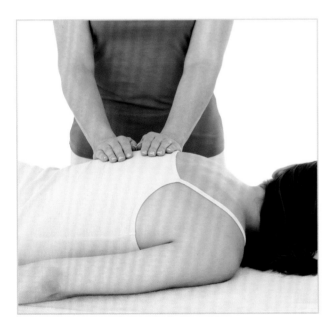

4 Now repeat Steps 2 and 3, starting with your hands one hand-width further down the back, treating the upper back.

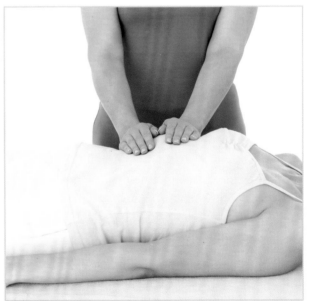

5 Additionally, treat the liver and gallbladder from the front, by placing your hands next to each other on the lower ribs and waist on the right side, in Front Position Two.

Middle- and lower-back pain

The most common causes of middle- and lower-back pain are low kidney function, poor dietary habits, stress and tension. Stress can disrupt the energy in the back muscles, which go into spasm when the kidneys and related lower-back muscles weaken. Pain in the middle back is associated with imbalance in the liver and spleen. Back pain can develop through heavy lifting, prolonged standing, lack of exercise, poor posture, reproductive problems and menstrual pain, but it can also be associated with a general lack of adequate support in life.

Recommended: Try to find the source of the back pain. If possible, alleviate the source of muscle tension, such as lack of exercise, excess sitting, stress and repressed emotions (for example, anger and fear). Change your posture in jobs that involve sitting and repetitive actions.

Treatment

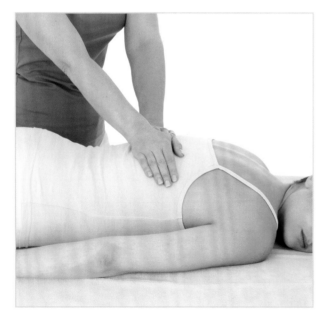

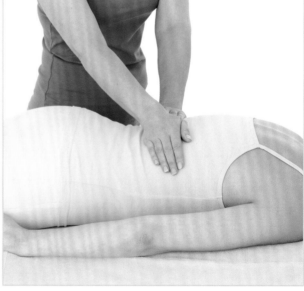

1 Lay both hands on the back, on the lower ribs above the waist, so that your hands cover the adrenal glands and the upper part of the kidneys.

2 Then move your hands down (one hand-width) to cover the kidneys at waist level, in Back Position Three. (Both Steps 1 and 2 help to balance the functions of the adrenals, kidneys and nervous system.)

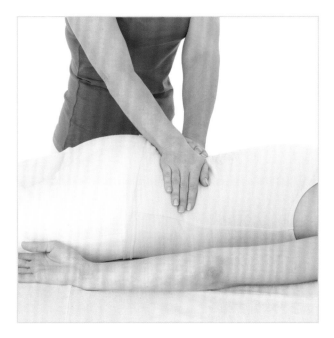

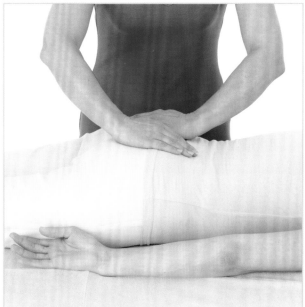

3 Place your hands on the lower part of the back at hip level, in Back Position Four.

4 Rest your hands on either side of the lower spine, over the sacrum: one hand with fingertips pointing down to the tailbone and the other hand pointing upwards. This relieves lower-back pain as well as helping sciatica, and strengthens the lymph and nerves.

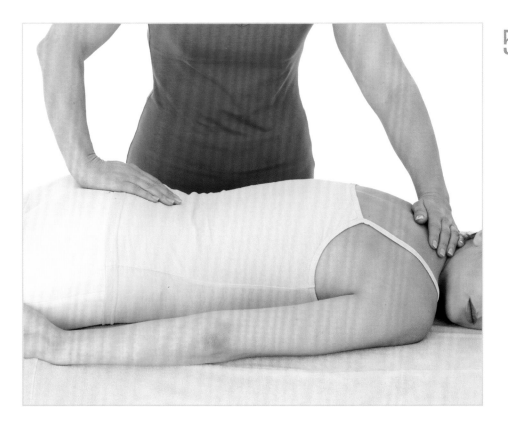

5 Complete the treatment by placing one hand on the coccyx and the other at the top of the spine on the neck. This balances the energy of the whole back, down the spine (see page 144). In addition, you can use the hand positions for treating the sciatic nerve: lay one hand directly on one buttock or over the sacrum, and the other on the heel on the same side (see page 144). Alternatively, you can treat the entire back using all the back positions (see page 138).

Sciatica

The sciatic nerve starts at waist level on both sides of the spine and runs down though the buttocks and legs. Sciatica generally occurs when a nerve becomes trapped by surrounding muscles. It can cause great pain and is sometimes accompanied by a tingling or numbness in the legs. However, holding back emotions or feeling unsupported in life can also contribute. All the following hand positions help to release sciatic pain in the lower back and legs.

Recommended: Carry on using Reiki, but also seek chiropractic treatment.

CASE STUDY
SCIATICA, BACK AND LEG PAIN

CLIENT PROFILE
Yvonne had a slipped disc and a two-year-old injury to her lower back, plus sciatica, and her right leg felt numb.

THE REIKI TREATMENT
After receiving Reiki (Back Position Four and Five and Buttocks, Legs and Heels Position, see page 144), the stiffness and pain in her right leg disappeared. With each treatment she commented on the feeling and aliveness coming back to her leg, and said she felt more refreshed and energized.

Treatment

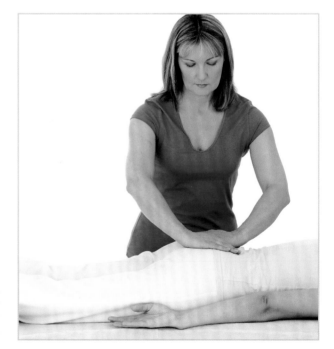

1 Place one hand over the sacral bone with the fingertips pointing downwards, and the other hand beside it, fingertips pointing upwards.

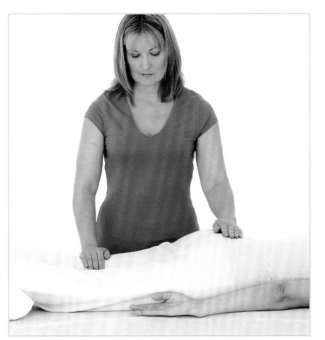

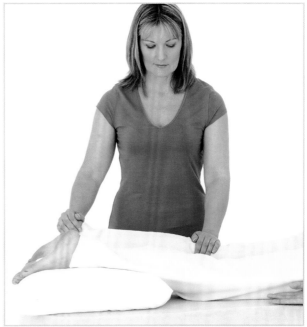

2 Lay one hand on the buttocks, where the pain is located, or place the hand over the sacrum. With the other hand, move down the leg, one hand-width at a time, on the same side, until you reach the knee. (See also the Buttocks, Legs and Heels Position, page 144.)

3 Keep one hand on the knee, and using the other hand, work your way down the leg, one hand-width at a time, to the heel.

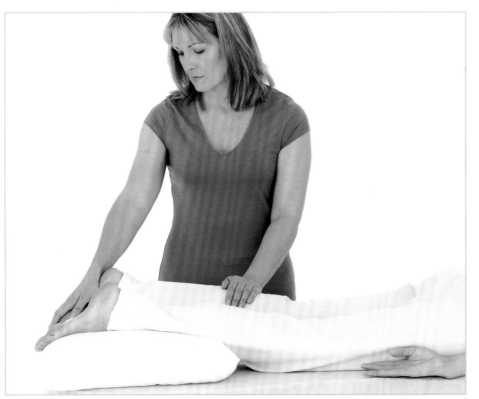

4 Lay one hand on the sole of the foot and the other hand just below the knee. Then treat the leg on the less painful side in the same way.

Colds and flu

Colds are infections in the mouth, nose and throat caused by viruses, and symptoms include sneezing, running nose, nasal congestion, cough, sore throat and headache. A cold is a natural way for the body to cleanse and detoxify itself of accumulated waste. Flu has similar symptoms to the common cold. It is characterized by head and muscle aches, as well as fever and chills, and is caused by various viruses. Similar to a cold, flu is the body's way of eliminating waste and toxins. Poor diet, stress and lack of exercise weaken the immune system, providing opportunity for viruses to work in the body.

Recommended (colds): Rest and drink plenty of fluids to support detoxification. Avoid taking medication to reduce or suppress symptoms, as this may stop the body's self-cleansing process. However, taking vitamin C and perhaps multivitamins can help to relieve symptoms.

Recommended (flu): Keep warm, rest in bed and keep the lighting low. Drink plenty of fluids (water or herbal teas) and listen to your body's needs. This is a time to relax, retreat and respect the demands of your body. If necessary, take the recommended pain relief, nasal decongestants, steam inhalation and throat lozenges to reduce the symptoms.

Treatment

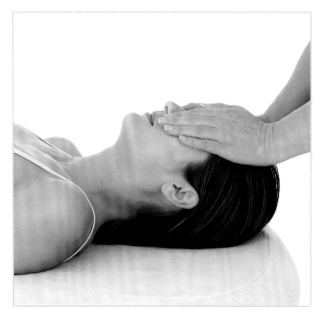

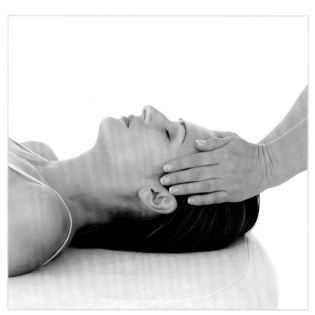

1 Lay your hands to the right and left of the nose, covering the forehead, eyes and cheeks, in Head Position One. This position helps the sinuses to clear out any blockage.

2 Then place your hands on both sides of the head above the ears, fingertips touching the temples, and palms following the curve of the head, in Head Position Two.

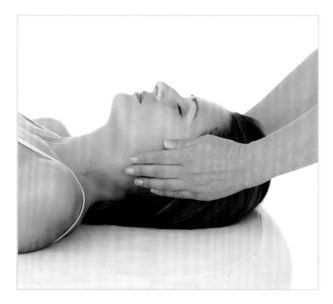

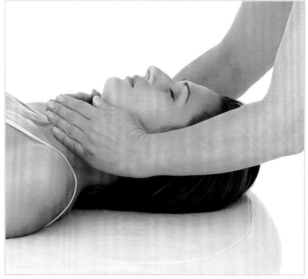

3 Place your hands over the ears, in Head Position Three. This helps to release any pressure in the inner ear and frees blockages, thus helping to relieve any disorders of the nose and throat and alleviating colds and flu.

4 Place your hands gently over either side of the throat, without touching it directly, in Head Position Five. This position treats the lymph nodes and eases sore throats and flu.

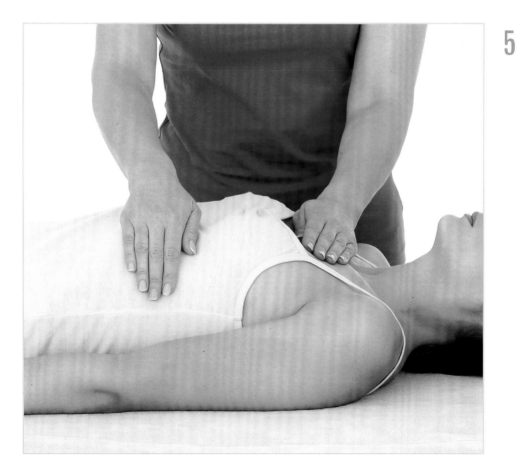

5 Lay your left hand on the lower left side of the ribcage (spleen area) and your right hand below the collarbone across the thymus gland. This position treats the lymphatic system and the spleen; it helps with problems of the immune system and supports detoxification. (See also the Spleen and Thymus-Gland Position, page 142.) Alternatively, you can give a full-body treatment or do self-treatment (see pages 134 and 128).

Coughs

Coughs are caused by dust, smoke, gases and inflammation of the upper airways, and are a side-effect of the common cold. Coughing is a reflex action to clear the throat of phlegm, mucus and other irritants. A persistent cough needs to be investigated by a medical doctor, as it indicates an underlying problem; in some cases medication is prescribed.

Recommended: Cut out dairy products, which cause an accumulation of mucus in the system.

Treatment

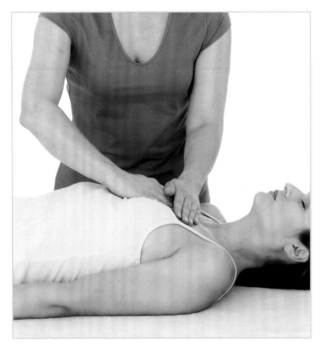

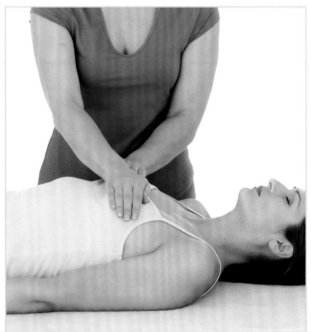

1 Place one hand horizontally on the middle of the chest and the other horizontally next to it beneath the collarbone. This position treats the upper lungs and thymus gland.

2 Lay your hands on the breasts or chest. If the receiver does not want their breasts touched, keep your hands 2.5 cm (1 in) above; Reiki energy is absorbed though the aura. (See also the Breast and Chest Position, page 142). This position treats the lungs.

Bronchitis

Bronchitis is an infection of the bronchi (air tubes leading from the windpipe to the lungs), accompanied by frequent coughing, which produces phlegm. This is caused by airborne organisms in the bronchi. The main causes of chronic bronchitis are smoking and pollution. It can also result from repeated suppression of colds through antibiotics or other medication.

Recommended: Stop smoking (passive and active) and drink plenty of fluids. Try steam inhalations, and use medication if necessary.

Treatment

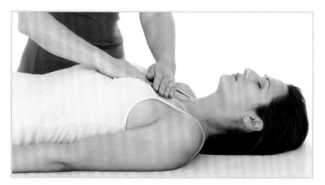

1 Place one hand horizontally on the middle of the chest and the other horizontally next to it beneath the collarbone. This position treats the upper lungs and thymus gland.

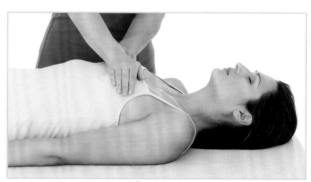

2 Lay your hands on the breasts or chest. If the receiver does not want their breasts touched, keep your hands 2.5 cm (1 in) above; Reiki energy is absorbed through the aura.

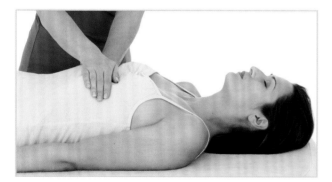

3 Continue by laying your hands one hand-width lower than the breast (above waist level), with one hand on the right side and the other on the left side, so that the fingers of one hand touch the base of the other. This strengthens the immune system and supports the respiratory tract.

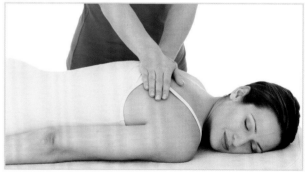

4 Place both hands on the upper back between the shoulder blades, one hand on each side of the body, with the fingertips of one hand touching the spine and the base of the other hand, in Back Position Two. This position is good for lung disorders, coughs and bronchitis.

Asthma

Asthma is a recurrent inflammation of the bronchi and bronchioles. A history of chronic colds and bronchitis often precedes its onset. The inflammation causes constriction and increases the production of phlegm, which narrows the air passages. Symptoms are breathlessness, wheezing and coughing. Asthma often develops in childhood and resolves later in life. Attacks can be triggered by exercise, infection, pollen, dust, stress and an intake of high doses of antibiotics, which weaken the auto-immune system. There can be a connection between weak kidneys and the onset of symptoms.

Recommended: Eliminate wheat, sugar and dairy products from your diet. Try cutting out animal protein to cleanse the system. Also avoid coffee, tea and alcohol.

Treatment

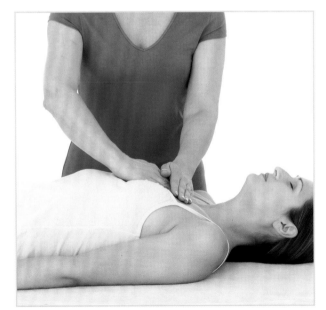

1 Place one hand horizontally across the thymus gland (below the collarbone) and the other at right angles to the first, in the middle of the chest, in Front Position One.

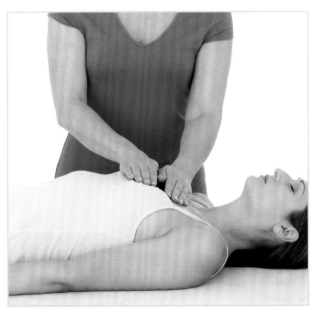

2 Place one hand horizontally on the middle of the chest and the other, also horizontally, on the breastbone, below the collarbone. This position treats the upper lungs and the thymus gland.

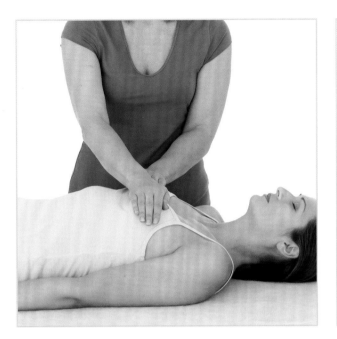

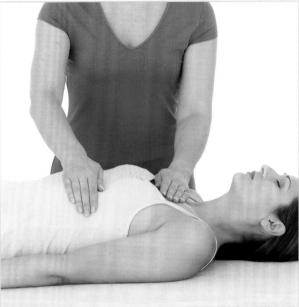

3 Lay your hands on the receiver's breast/chest. If the receiver does not want their breasts touched, hold your hands 2.5 cm (1 in) above. This position treats the lungs.

4 Place one hand on the thymus gland (horizontally on the upper breastbone), below the collarbone, and lay the other hand on the spleen area on the left side of the body, on the lower ribcage.

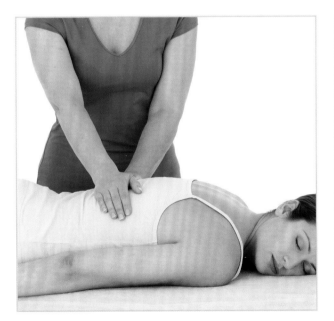

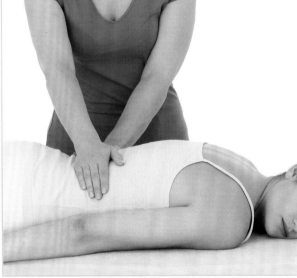

5 Place both hands on the back over the lower ribs above the waist, so that your hands cover the adrenal glands and the upper part of the kidneys.

6 Then move your hands down (by one hand-width) to cover the kidneys at waist level, in Back Position Three. This helps balance the functions of the adrenals, kidneys and nervous system.

Allergies

An allergy is a condition with an inappropriate immune response triggered by contact with an otherwise harmless substance, such as dust, pollen or other airborne particles. Allergic reactions can also result from ingestion of a particular food and from skin contact with chemicals. Often the liver is unable to neutralize certain substances, causing a build-up and an immune reaction. The substance that the body recognizes as 'foreign' accumulates in places such as the lymph system, intestine, liver and spleen. The immune system tends to overwork to rid the body of the substances, which can suffer a total breakdown in consequence. Use this sequence for hay fever, skin and food allergies and all other allergies.

Recommended: Drink a minimum of 2 litres (3½ pints) of still water per day to help the detoxification process. In addition, you might want to try homeopathy; use a ginger compress on the liver to eliminate toxins; or try singing to strengthen the spleen, as this is the allergy-fighting organ. With regards to food, avoid the substance to which you are allergic. Refined sugar, wheat, vinegar and milk products can trigger an allergy.

CASE STUDY **ECZEMA**

CLIENT PROFILE
When the baby son of Maria (a Third Degree Reiki trainee) had his first injection, he developed a very large boil on his leg and the start of eczema behind his knees. Doctors denied it could have anything to do with the injection and wanted his mother to give him antibiotics; she refused. The eczema spread all over his body and would weep and bleed.

THE REIKI TREATMENT
As well as altering his diet, his mother decided to give him Reiki for about 10–15 minutes per day, mainly using the hand positions 'Self-balancing the Chakras' on pages 48–49. Three weeks later the baby stopped scratching overnight. From then on, his skin got better and better, and today is how it should be – beautiful.

Treatment

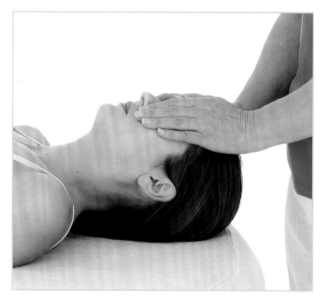

1 Lay your hands to the right and left of the nose, covering the forehead, eyes and cheeks, in Head Position One. This helps the sinuses to clear out any blockages.

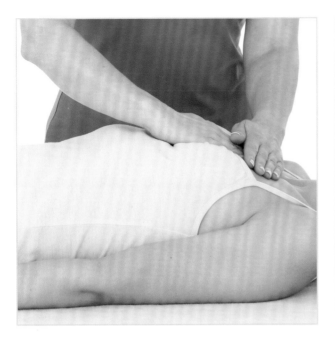

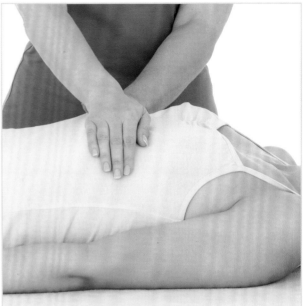

2 Place one hand horizontally across the thymus gland (below the collarbone) and the other at right angles to the first in the middle of the chest, in Front Position One. This treats the lungs and supports the immune system.

3 Lay your hands on the front on each side at waist level. This position treats the lymphatic system and helps clear toxins in the body.

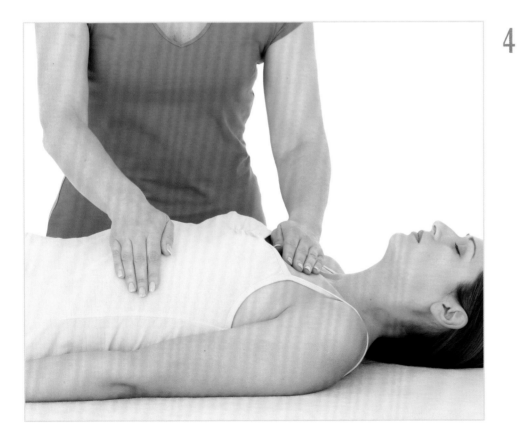

4 Place one hand on the thymus gland (horizontally on the upper breastbone) beneath the collarbone, and the other on the spleen area on the left side of the body on the lower ribcage. This position strengthens the immune system. Additionally, spend time working on the skin if there is a rash and also treat the liver, spleen, stomach and small and large intestines.

Arthritis

Arthritis is inflammation of a joint. Its symptoms are swelling, pain, redness and stiffness. There are three main forms: osteoarthritis, rheumatoid arthritis and infective arthritis. Osteoarthritis relates primarily to age and results from long-term wear and tear on the joints. Rheumatoid arthritis is an auto-immune disorder, where the body 'attacks' the joint; it usually affects the hands, wrists, feet and arms. Infective arthritis is an infection of the joint fluids, caused by bacteria; it can be related to infections such as mumps, rheumatic fever, rubella or chickenpox.

Recommended: Avoid eating dairy produce and animal fats. You might need to take medication. Do some gentle exercise and get to know about dietary supplements that will help the joints.

CASE STUDY **ARTHRITIS**

CLIENT PROFILE
Lorna (a Second Degree Reiki trainee) had suffered from inflammation, swelling and pain in the joints. Usually the pain appeared over a period of time – three days – and always affected a different area/joint in the body, and then disappeared for a month or so.

THE REIKI TREATMENT
One night she had severe and almost unbearable pain in her left shoulder. She had no pain killers and was giving Reiki to herself over one hour, directly on the spot of pain (cupping the left shoulder with her right hand). Even after 15 minutes she felt the pain slowly subsiding. The next morning she had no pain at all and felt much better.

Treatment

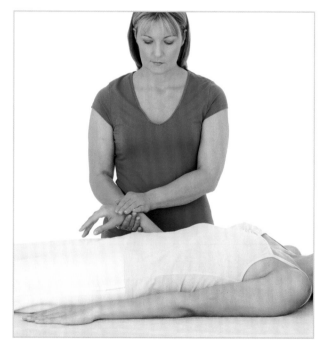

1 Treat the joints with the 'sandwich' position: place one hand above and the other below the area; or treat it sideways (with one hand on one side, and the other hand on the other side).

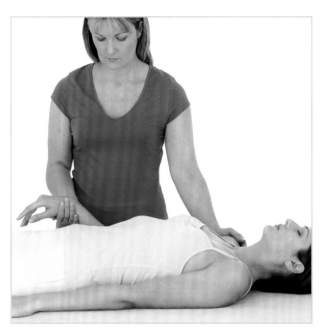

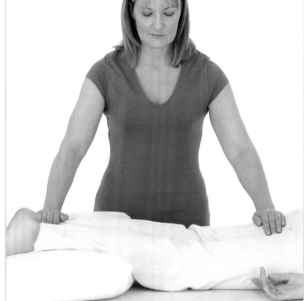

2 Additionally, let energy flow through the arms, legs and feet. Place one hand at the top of the shoulder area and the other on the wrist. Keep your hands in position until you feel that the energy is balanced.

3 Place one hand on the upper leg where it joins the buttocks, and the other hand at the ankle, letting energy flow in the leg.

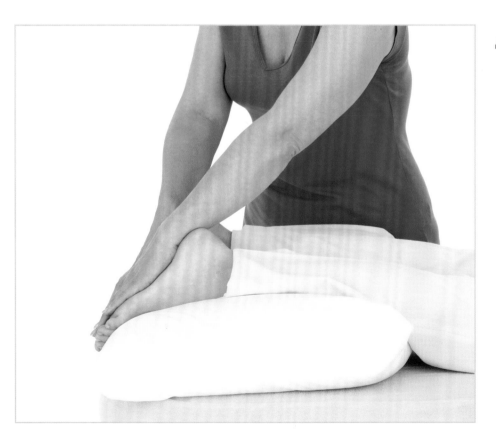

4 Lay one hand on the sole of each foot, with the fingertips covering the toes, in Sole Position (A). This is good for treating the foot reflex zones of the whole body. Alternatively, give a full Reiki treatment (see page 134) and spend extra time on the area where the pain is felt.

Insomnia and sleep problems

Insomnia is a disturbance to regular sleep patterns; sufferers find it hard to fall asleep or to remain asleep. This may be related to environmental factors (noise and light) or lifestyle (too much caffeine, lack of exercise, irregular sleep patterns). Physical causes, such as hormonal disturbances (during the menopause), need to be investigated, as does an excessive period of insomnia, which can have a serious underlying problem such as anxiety, depression or drug withdrawal. Insomnia due to worry is common. Symptoms include fatigue, irritability and difficulty in coping with daily tasks.

Recommended: Try not to eat later than 3–4 hours before going to sleep. Generally avoid coffee, sweets (especially before bed), black tea and soft drinks. Establishing regular rituals before going to bed – such as reading, going for a short walk, a little exercise (perhaps yoga) and keeping the bedroom aired – can all help in developing regular sleeping patterns. If necessary, try herbal remedies, which can be used over a period of time.

Treatment

1 Lay your hands, with your index fingers touching, to the right and left of the nostrils, covering the forehead, eyes and cheeks, in Head Position One. This balances the pituitary and pineal glands, which govern hormonal balance in the body. This position is good for exhaustion and stress, and affects the whole body.

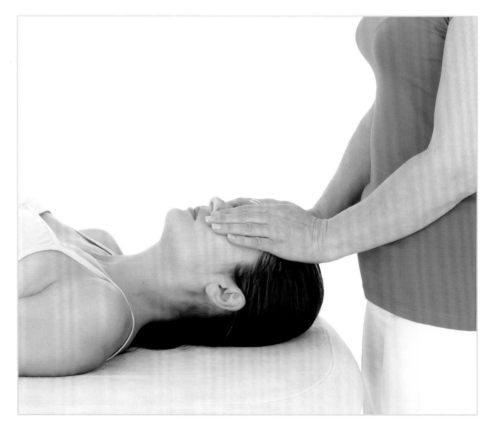

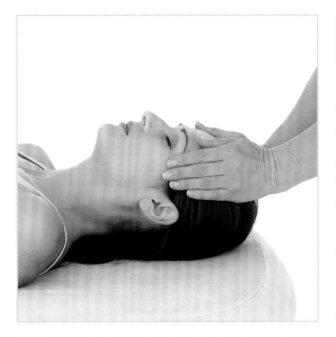

2 Place your hands on both sides of the head, above the ears, fingertips touching the temples, and palms following the curve of the head, in Head Position Two. This balances the right and left sides of the brain, helps to ease stress and excessive mental activity, and calms the mind.

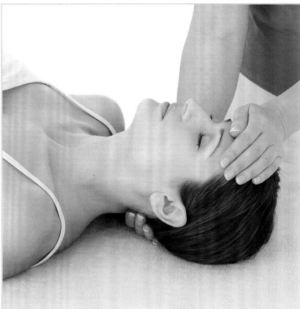

3 Lay one hand on the back of the head over the medulla oblongata and the other over the forehead (third-eye chakra). This position reduces stress, facilitates meditation and helps sleeping problems.

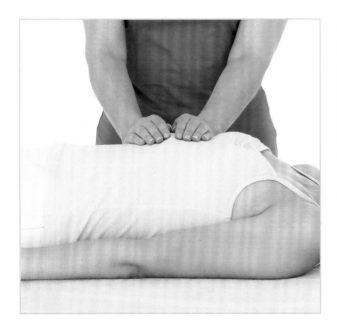

4 Lay one hand on the lower ribcage on the right side, below the chest, with the other hand directly below it at waist level, in Front Position Two. This position treats the liver and gallbladder, and also balances emotions such as anger and depression.

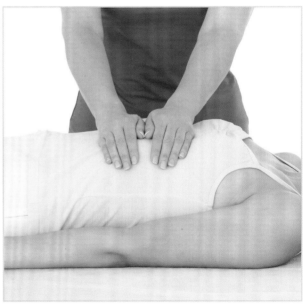

5 Treat the opposite side (left side) in the same way, in Front Position Three. This is good for digestive disorders and helps stabilize the immune system.

Cystitis

Cystitis is inflammation of the bladder and is caused by bacterial growths on the bladder wall. Symptoms are frequent urination accompanied by a burning sensation, with pain in the bladder area. Even if the bladder is emptied, there may be still a desire to pass urine. This condition is most common in women, because the urethral opening is much shorter than it is in men. In men, cystitis usually occurs because of urine retention.

Recommended: Drink large quantities of water to help flush out the bacteria. Medication can also be prescribed. Avoid highly acidic food, such as meat, dairy products, eggs, citrus fruit, refined sugar, oily food, salt, caffeine, alcohol and spicy food. Drink lots of spring water, herbal teas and cranberry, carrot and lemon juices. Meditate and rest to restore harmony and balance to the body.

The treatment sequence can also be used for bed-wetting and incontinence.

CASE STUDY **CYSTITIS**

CLIENT PROFILE
Isabelle suffered from chronic cystitis and kidney complaints, which became acute a few times a year.

THE REIKI TREATMENT
She was treated with Reiki (Front Position Five and over the pubic bone and reproductive area – see the treatment positions for cystitis below and opposite) when she was in great pain, and later that day reported that she felt much better.

Treatment

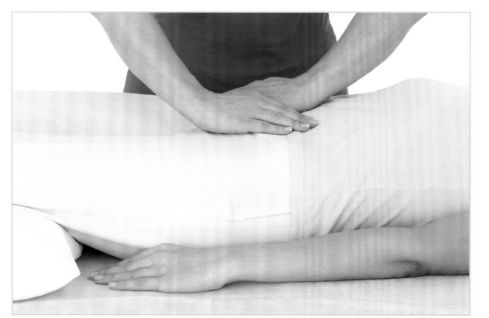

1 Place both hands on the pubic bone over the reproductive area. One hand should be pointing down, the other pointing up. If the receiver feels uncomfortable being touched here, keep your hands just above the area; Reiki energy is absorbed through the receiver's aura.

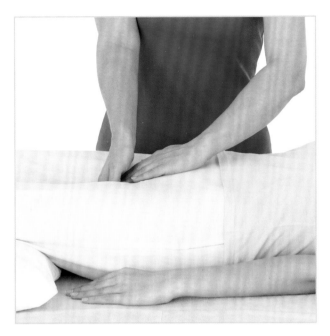

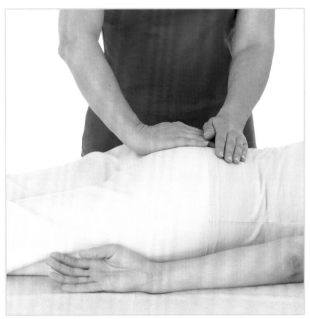

2 Lay one hand over the pubic area and the other between the legs, with the palm of the hand tight over the reproductive area. Ask the receiver beforehand if they feel comfortable being touched here.

3 Place one hand across the sacrum (on the lower back) and the other at right angles to the first, over the coccyx, to form a T-shape. This position helps bladder disorders.

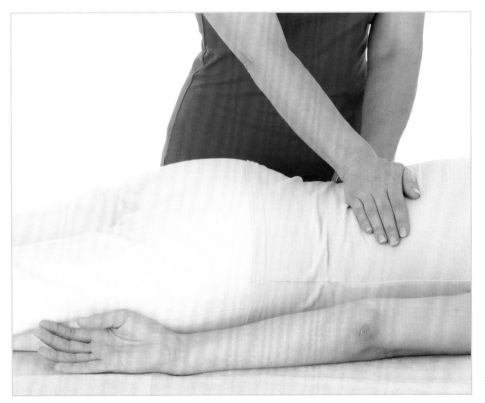

4 Additionally, treat the kidneys: lay your hands on the lower ribs, above the kidneys, using Back Position Three; also treat the adrenals, moving your hands one hand-width higher than Back Position Three.

Indigestion (dyspepsia)

Indigestion is experienced as heartburn, abdominal pain, nausea or flatulence. It is usually caused by eating too quickly or too much, or overly rich or spicy food. It may also be caused by stress. Other reasons can be emotional upsets and poor food combinations, or an imbalance in the spleen, the organ that supplies life-force energy to the small and large intestines. It is important that the spleen is not weakened by a poor diet.

Recommended: Develop healthy eating habits. Eat simple meals and try to combine food such as protein with leafy green vegetables. Protein and carbohydrate (starch) should be eaten at separate meals. Fruits and sweetened foods should be eaten on their own. The following foods aid digestion: apples, barley, grapefruit peel, lemons, limes and carrots. Avoid meat, dairy products, eggs, poor-quality oils, sugar, spicy food, fried food and alcohol.

Treatment

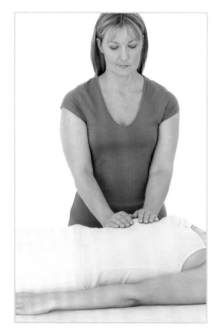 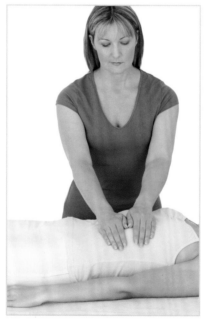 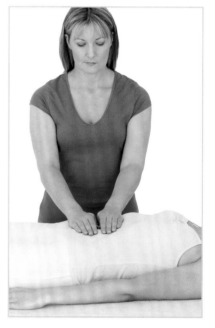

1 Lay your hands next to each other on the receiver's lower ribs and waist on the right side, in Front Position Two. This treats the digestive areas (pancreas, duodenum, liver, gallbladder, stomach and large intestine).

2 Then place both hands on the left side in the same way, in Front Position Three. This treats the spleen and pancreas, and is good for digestive disorders.

3 Additionally, place one hand above the navel (solar-plexus area) and the other below the navel, in Front Position Four. This treats the stomach and intestines, and eases bloated feelings.

Diarrhoea

Diarrhoea is the passing of frequent, watery faeces, usually caused by eating contaminated food. Chronic diarrhoea may be an indication of underlying disease, for example Crohn's disease, ulcerative colitis or irritable bowel syndrome, but in most cases it is due to a weakness in the digestive system; this includes the spleen, stomach, pancreas, liver, gallbladder and small and large intestines. Diarrhoea can be viewed as the body's normal reaction to the presence of a toxin in the digestive tract. It is a way for the body to eliminate viruses, bacteria and toxic food. The main concern is the loss of body fluids, minerals and salts. In children, diarrhoea can be dangerous and should always be referred urgently to a medical doctor.

Recommended: Drink plenty of water and add minerals and salt to your drinks. Avoid certain foods, such as honey, spinach, cow's milk, apricots, plums, sesame seeds and any food that is difficult to digest. Consider consulting a qualified homeopath for further help. Use meditation and massage for deep relaxation.

Treatment

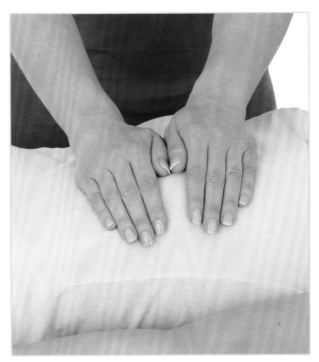

1 Use all three hand positions as for indigestion (see the instructions opposite).

CASE STUDY **CROHN'S DISEASE**

CLIENT PROFILE
Regina had been suffering from Crohn's disease of the large intestine for many years, and was taking steroids on a continuous basis.

THE REIKI TREATMENT
After having had a few full Reiki treatments, using all the 17 basic hand positions (see pages 134–140), with extra time spent on Front Positions Two–Five, she no longer needed steroids and her pain was gone. Her medical specialist was delighted with her progress.

Constipation

Constipation can be described as the passing of hard, dry, infrequent faeces. Symptoms such as a headache, coated tongue, sense of tiredness, bad breath and depression often accompany constipation. A lack of fibre in the diet and a weakness of the spleen can also be the cause.

Recommended: Eat a high-fibre diet, consisting of green leafy vegetables and wholegrains. Eat plenty of raw fruit. Drink plenty of water (2–3 litres/3½–5 pints) per day. Perhaps use acupuncture (or acupressure) to strengthen the meridians of the spleen. Do some regular stretching and yoga exercises, and take daily brisk walks.

Treatment

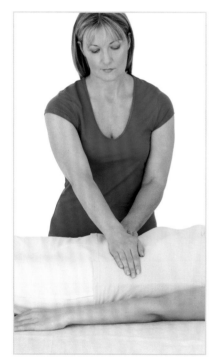 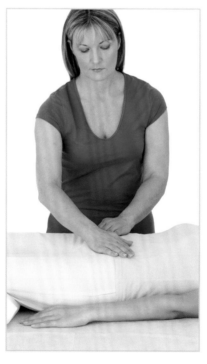 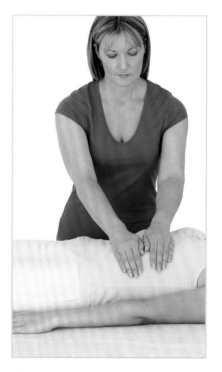

1 Place your hands at waist level and around the navel on the front side, so that the base of one palm touches the fingertips of the other. This treats the large intestine and any intestinal disorders.

2 Continue treating the colon area and lay your hands in a V-shape (one hand pointing down, the other pointing up) over the pubic area, using Front Position Five.

3 Additionally, place both hands on the left side of the body over the lower ribs at waist level, using Front Position Three. This treats the spleen and pancreas, and is good for digestive disorders.

Irritable bowel syndrome

The symptoms of irritable bowel syndrome (IBS) are cramping, abdominal pain, bloating, constipation and diarrhoea. This can cause a great deal of discomfort and distress, although it does not permanently harm the intestines and does not lead to serious disease such as cancer. Most people can control the symptoms with diet, stress management and prescribed medication. For some people, however, IBS can be disabling and they may be unable to work, travel or attend social occasions. Sometimes people find that their symptoms subside for a few months and then return, while others suffer a constant worsening of symptoms over time.

Recommended: Avoid large meals, wheat, rye, barley, chocolate, milk products, alcohol and drinks with caffeine, such as coffee, tea and cola. Avoid stress and emotional upsets, as well as conflicting situations. Allergy testing is recommended, as people with IBS might not be able to digest gluten, which is found in wheat, rye and barley. People with coeliac disease, which can be determined by a blood test, cannot eat these foods.

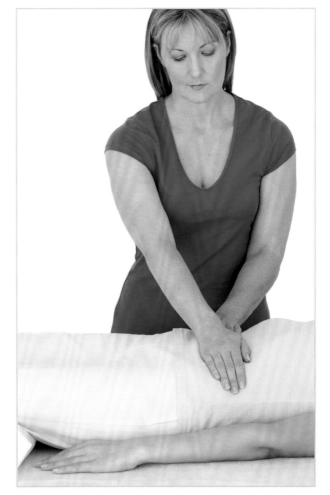

Treatment

1 Use all three hand positions as for indigestion (see page 186). This treatment also works for flatulence, a build-up of gas in the digestive tract that may result from IBS, indigestion or gallbladder disorders.

Menstrual problems

Some women suffer more than others from menstrual and premenstrual problems. Painful periods (dysmenorrhoea) are common and the reasons are unknown, while amenorrhoea (absence of periods) occurs because of stress, starvation, anorexia and pregnancy. Excessive bleeding (menorrhagia) may be a result of a hormonal imbalance, inter-uterine contraceptives, fibroids or polyps (tissue growths). Changes to normal periods can indicate an underlying problem. Any menstruation problems should be investigated by a medical doctor, who will check out irregularities in the cycle. Women with premenstrual syndrome symptoms, such as breast tenderness, imbalanced periods and heavy bleeding, usually have high oestrogen levels.

Recommended: Avoid eating red meat, too much salt in foods, sugar, dairy fats and caffeine. Taking supplements such as vitamin B complex, C and E, as well as calcium, magnesium and zinc, can help the symptoms. Avoid emotional stress and do abdominal exercise to strengthen the uterus. Consider homeopathy or the use of essential oils. You might want to explore emotional issues such as: what are your deepest feelings about being a woman?

CASE STUDY **MENSTRUAL PAIN**

CLIENT PROFILE
Catherine (a First Degree Reiki trainee) used to get cramps and feel tired during her period.

THE REIKI TREATMENT
She has felt much better since she started herself on Reiki (using the self-treatment Front Positions Three and Four, page 130, laying hands directly on the spot of pain). The pain in her abdomen is much less severe when she gives herself Reiki; she feels a lot of heat coming through her hands and it really helps to calm the cramping.

Treatment

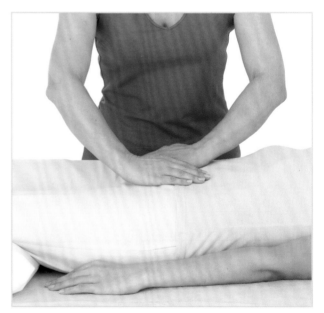

1 Place both hands on the pubic bone over the reproductive area. One hand should be pointing down, the other pointing up. If the receiver feels uncomfortable being touched here, keep your hands just above the area; Reiki energy is absorbed through the receiver's aura.

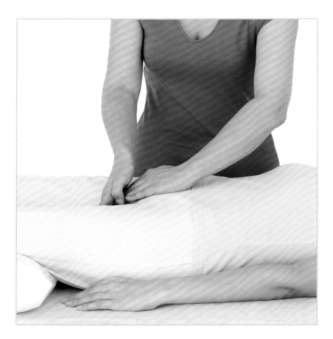

2 Lay one hand over the pubic area and the other between the legs, with the palm of the hand tight over the reproductive area. Ask the receiver beforehand if they feel comfortable being touched here.

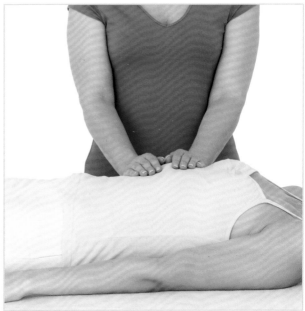

3 Lay your hands next to each other on the receiver's lower ribs and waist on the right side, in Front Position Two.

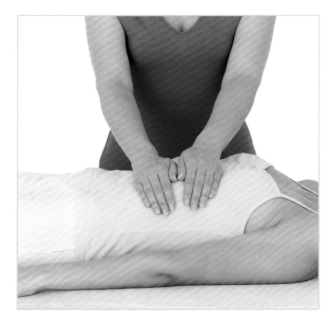

4 Now place both hands on the left side in the same way, in Front Position Three. Both positions treat the bowel and digestive areas.

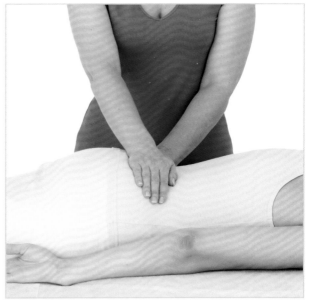

5 To ease any back pain, go directly to the pain area and place your hands on the lower back at hip level, in Back Position Four.

6 Place one hand across the sacrum and the other at right angles to the first, over the coccyx, cupping the buttocks, in Back Position Five (A) – T Position.

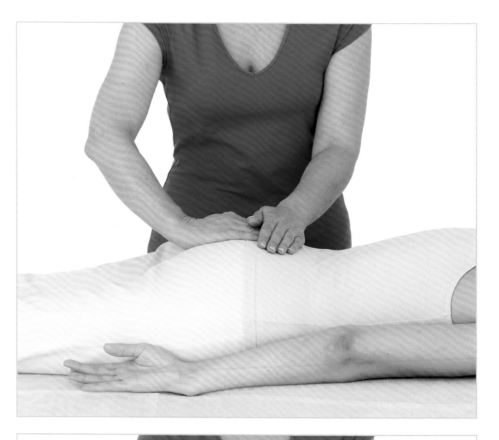

7 Additionally, place your hands, one pointing down and one pointing up, directly on the area where the pain is, over the pubic bone, in Front Position Five.

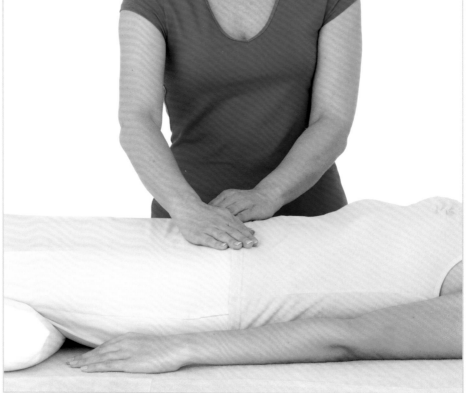

Menopause

Menopause is the cessation of menstruation in women due to major changes in the hormonal balance, and usually occurs between the mid-forties and -fifties. Symptoms include 'hot flushes', vaginal dryness, disturbed sleeping patterns, night sweats, moodiness, memory lapses, aching joints, decreased interest in sex and depression. Osteoporosis (increased bone brittleness) and raised fat levels in the blood can also occur. In traditional cultures it is seen as the 'peak' of womanhood, but in Western society it can be an emotionally charged time, and women may need to open new doors to find fresh levels of self-discovery. Medical doctors tend to prescribe hormone-replacement therapy (HRT), which can lead to a higher risk of unwanted body fat, water retention and even cancer.

Recommended: It is important to eat a healthy diet low in fat and high in fibre. Avoid eating meat, animal protein and fat, sugar and refined foods. Coffee and alcohol can cause hot flushes; instead eat more fresh fish, fruit and vegetables. It is also beneficial to take suitable nutritional supplements (consult a nutritionist). Do physical exercise and stretches on a regular basis, such as brisk daily walks, cycling, dancing, Tai Chi and yoga. Some women benefit from complementary treatments – homeopathy, Chinese herbal treatments and Bach Flower Remedies.

Treatment

1 Place both hands on the pubic bone over the reproductive area. One hand should be pointing down, the other pointing up. If the receiver feels uncomfortable being touched here, position your hands just above the area instead.

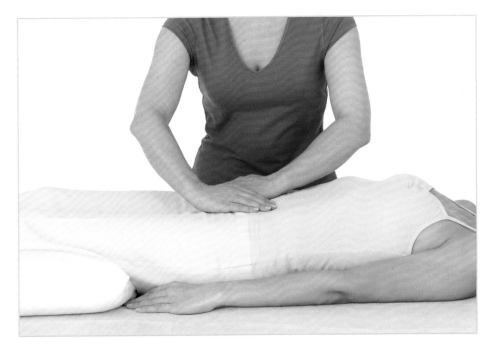

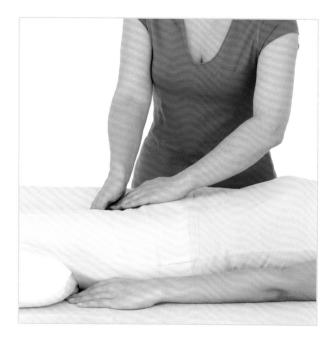

2 Lay one hand over the pubic area and the other between the legs, with the palm of the hand tight over the reproductive area. Ask the receiver beforehand if they feel comfortable being touched here.

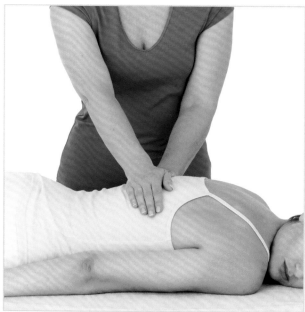

3 Place one hand on the left side of the back on the lower ribs above the waist (one hand-width lower than Back Position Two), with the fingertips touching the base of the other palm, which is placed opposite on the right side of the back.

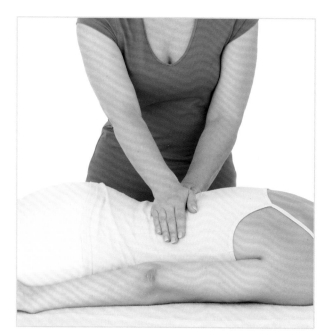

4 Move both hands one hand-width down, keeping your hands slightly above the waist. This treats the adrenal glands, which regulate the stress response, metabolism and sex drive.

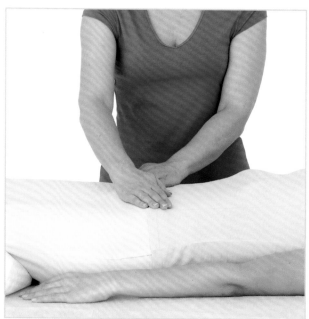

5 Place your hands over the pubic bone in the shape of a V, in Front Position Five, treating the female organs.

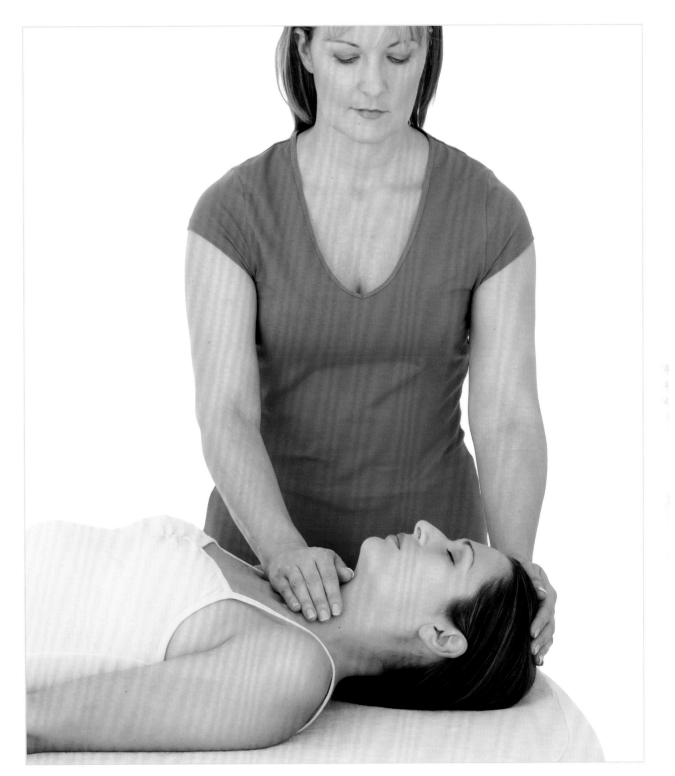

6 Additionally, lay one hand directly over the throat on the front, treating the thyroid (fifth chakra), and the other hand on the centre on the top of the head (seventh chakra). This treats the thyroid, pineal and pituitary glands, as well as the hypothalamus; it balances the metabolism and is helpful when experiencing weight problems.

Diabetes

Diabetes results from an inability of the pancreas to maintain normal blood-glucose levels. There are two types of diabetes: Type 1 arises when the pancreas produces only small amounts of insulin (or none). It is linked to a virus infection that causes the destruction of insulin-producing cells, and needs to be treated through insulin injections, diet and exercise.

Type 2 occurs when the pancreas produces minimal insulin, or when the cells are less receptive to the effects of insulin. It is related to age and obesity, and is treated through diet, exercise and in some cases with medication to stimulate insulin production. High levels of stress, adrenal exhaustion and prolonged demands (through poor dietary habits) on the pancreas and liver are the main causes of diabetes.

Recommended: Avoid stress and exhaustion. Eat a healthy diet containing lots of wholegrains and green vegetables, pulses, whole and cooked fruit, green beans, garlic, oatmeal and linseed oil. Avoid food that is rich in animal fat, dairy products, sugar, white flour and white rice. Regular daily walks (20–30 minutes) will improve the circulation, but avoid competitive sports.

Treatment

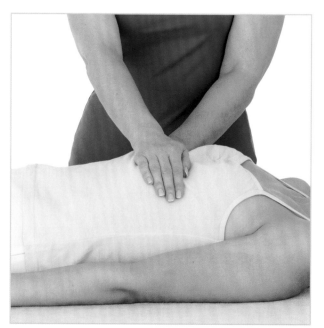

1 Place both hands beneath the breasts, with one hand under the breastbone on the right side and the other hand on the left side, so that the base of one palm is touching the fingertips of the other hand. This treats the pancreas.

2 Place your hands on the back, so that the base of one palm touches the fingertips of the other hand, one hand-width lower than Back Position Two (see page 131).

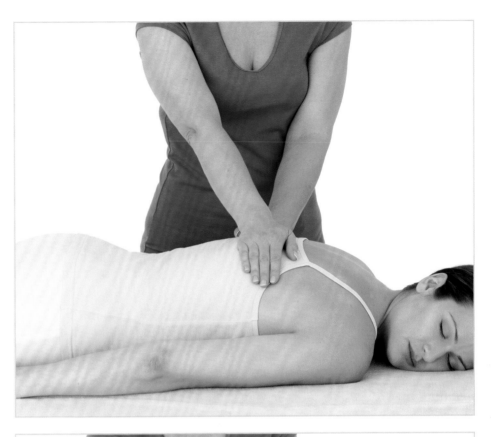

3 Move both hands down one hand-width from the previous position. Keep your hands slightly above the waist, with the base of one palm touching the fingertips of the other hand. Both positions treat the adrenal glands and upper part of the kidneys, which are important for releasing stress from the body.

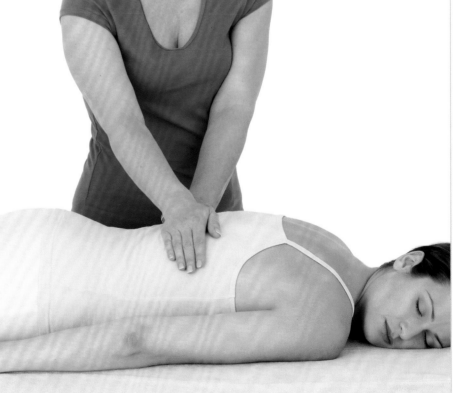

Earache and ear infection

Earache is a pain originating within the ear or its surrounding area. Infections occur in the middle ear, ear canal, bone at the rear of the ear or inner ear. Other forms of earache may be the result of pain that occurs in tonsillitis, flu, throat cancer, jaw and neck-muscle pain. A common cause of hearing problems in children is a persistent build-up of glue in the ear, stemming from an infection. A diet rich in mucus-forming foods (such as dairy products) can also bring about an ear infection. Tinnitus (a ringing sound in the ear) is an unpleasant disorder traditionally associated with old age, although nowadays younger people also suffer from it.

Recommended: Avoid eating wheat, dairy products, meat, hydrogenated oils and sugar. Instead eat carrots, lightly steamed vegetables, rice and citrus fruit, and drink carrot juice. Use tea-tree oil as an anti-inflammatory (massage it around the outer ear and neck area).

All positions treat the inner and outer ear and the organs of balance.

CASE STUDY **TINNITUS**

CLIENT PROFILE
Anna, aged 74 years, sought Reiki treatment because she had suffered from tinnitus for 14 years.

THE REIKI TREATMENT
After receiving a series of four Reiki sessions using the the full-body treatment, with particular attention to the head and ears (see Steps 1–5 right and opposite), she felt that the noise was slowly lessening, and after a further four treatments the noise disappeared totally during the daytime and sometimes during the night. She decided to learn Reiki herself and now gives herself at least one full treatment a day. Within eight weeks of starting these self-treatments, the tinnitus disappeared completely.

Treatment

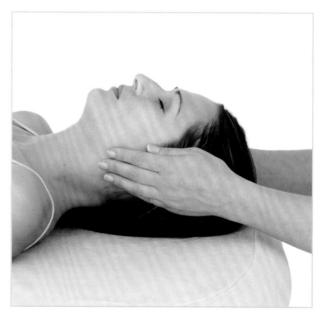

1 Place your hands over the ears on either side of the head, in Head Position Three. This helps disorders of the outer and inner ear, poor hearing and noises or hissing in the ears (tinnitus).

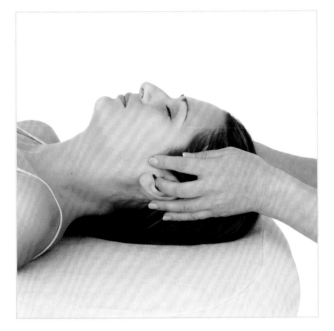

2 Place your middle finger gently on the ear opening (bending the middle finger). Lay the index finger on the head in front of the ear, and place the ring and little finger on the head behind the ear.

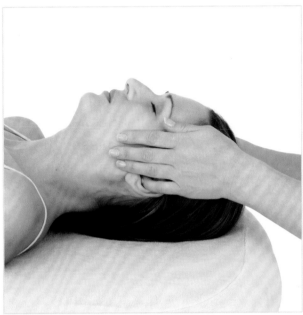

3 Alternatively, you can treat the ears directly by placing the little finger of each hand in the entrance of each ear.

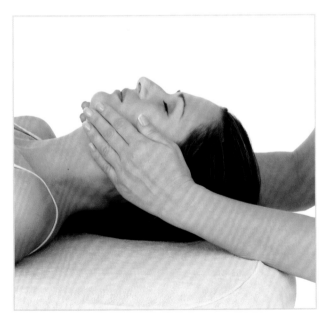

4 Place your hands either side of the jaw so that they cover the ears.

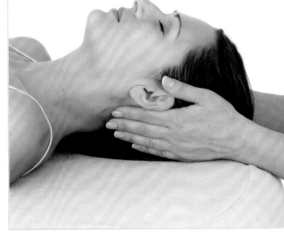

5 Additionally, place your palms behind the ears, with the thumbs above and slightly in front of the ears.

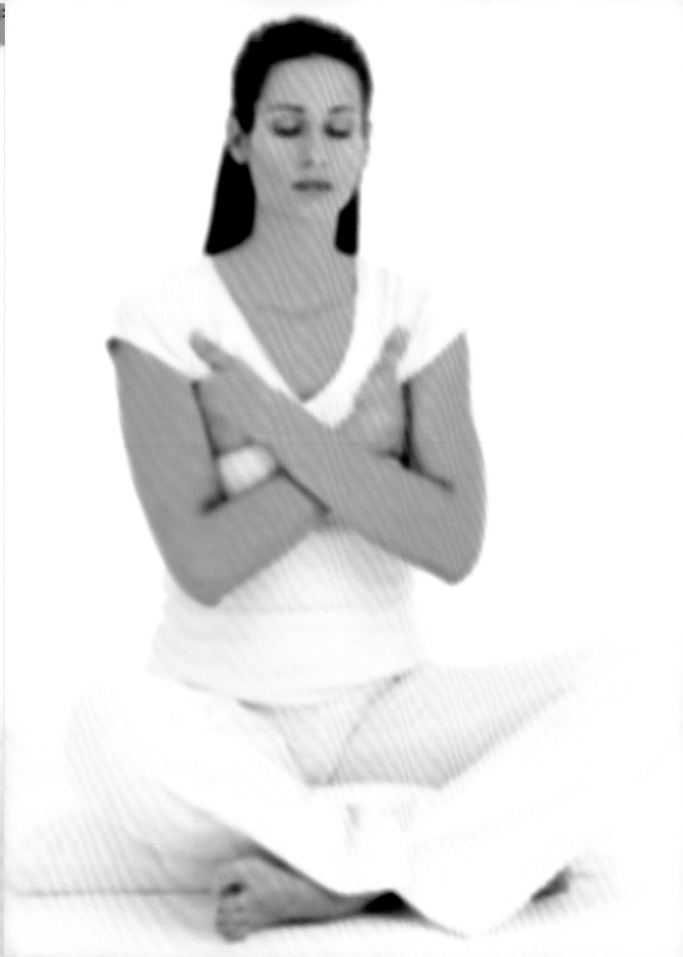

Reiki for healing the spirit

Reiki energy heals, harmonizes and balances the whole person: mind, body and spirit. This chapter is concerned with using Reiki to heal on a spiritual level. Here you will find different spiritual issues and themes, growth challenges, and the life stages everyone goes through to achieve their potential, wisdom and awareness, developing a loving and enjoyable relationship with yourself and with life itself. Finally, you can wake up to your own truth, to 'who you really are'.

Reiki as a spiritual discipline

The Usui system takes any 'sincere' Reiki Master on a lifelong journey: it is an art of living and healing. As each art requires discipline, so does the Reiki method. This particular discipline consists of faith, commitment, focus, patience, responsibility, honesty and self-control. Part of a Reiki Master's personal process is their spiritual development through Reiki as a lifelong practice. Any discipline that takes us to wholeness is a practice in which miracles of insight and transformation occur along the way, where we learn to accept everything that happens in life, whether wanted or unwanted, with humility and thankfulness.

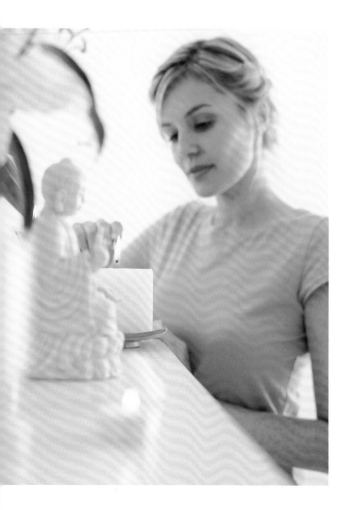

Spiritual healing

Reiki enables us to grow in spiritually creative ways, becoming aware of old energy patterns, belief systems, negative thought processes and behaviours that are obstacles to gaining personal freedom and self-realization. We need to heal ourselves and become 'whole' again, so that 'baggage' can dissolve, leaving us feeling alive and vital, enjoying a simple, fulfilling life.

Transforming toxic energy

When unexpected, unwelcome events occur – such as a redundancy, a separation or change in a relationship, a lost career, an unexpected relocation, reduced living standards or any other unsettling incident – we tend to react with strong negative emotions and vehemently oppose the change. After a while, perhaps we get tired of dwelling on the issue and believe we've 'got over' it. The truth is, in most cases, that we have merely stored this uncomfortable incident in the 'basement' of the mind, suppressing it, not wanting to be reminded of it any more. However, the energy of each 'poisoned' emotion is still there, held in the physical body (tissues, organs, muscles and bones). Such emotions are powerful and must not be underestimated; they are the real cause of

Reiki gives you the opportunity to develop spiritually, to heal and revitalize your thoughts and emotions, and to gain fresh insights. But it is a discipline that requires faith and focus.

'spiritual ill health'. Only the insight and determination to deal with these emotions in such a way that they can be turned into love, understanding and forgiveness can transform this toxic energy.

Taking back the power

We need to look at our lives as if we are a teacher. We need to be intelligent and understand life's messages to learn from our experiences. This has the potential of accessing new qualities in us, such as patience, understanding, tolerance, flexibility, courage and the readiness to let go or give up control. Life always runs more smoothly when we take conscious action for positive change, realizing that 'spiritual ill health' does not need to be our destiny, but can be a result of our negative thoughts and emotions. We take the power back into ourselves and know that we can make the right decisions in order to change life. This speeds up the healing process and supports a feeling of trust and strength in ourselves.

Daily practice

An important aspect of Reiki as a spiritual discipline is using it as a daily self-treatment practice. Meditating on and using the Reiki Principles (see pages 20–23) as guidelines for living is part of this. Masters 'draw' or visualize the Master Symbol (see page 118) with the intention for Reiki to fill their being all the time. This is a powerful contribution to your spiritual journey and contributes to your personal healing. The more you use Reiki, the more your energy channel is cleared and widened. You receive increased amounts of Universal Life Energy, so that through your expanded energy field other people are touched by that vibration. You can relax deeply and experience oneness. This is an ongoing process and an adventure with Reiki and yourself, spreading healing and harmony wherever you go. You experience the fullness of who you are: a divine being (spirit) having a precious human (physical) experience.

To aid you on your personal spiritual journey, it is important that you commit to the practice of daily self-treatment and meditation on the fundamental Reiki Principles.

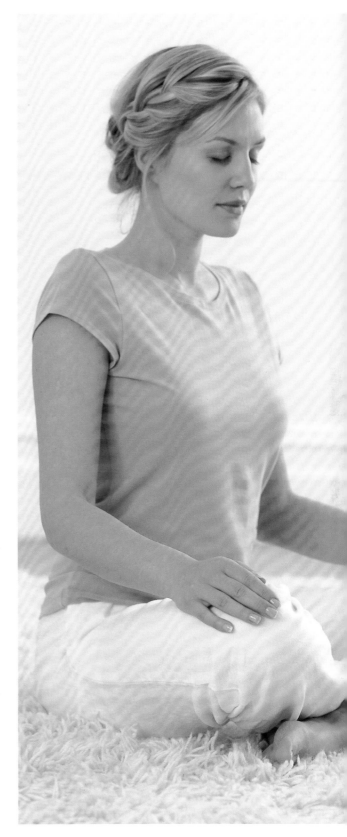

Meditation

Meditation is a state of being where we feel at one with each and every thing, which is an important tool in your Reiki life journey. We cannot 'make' this oneness happen; it just occurs by itself, when the mind is still and in meditation. Meditation techniques are a precise, scientific way to go deeper into the self by emptying yourself of everything that is not 'you'.

Inner-peace meditation

The heart is a natural source of peace. With this meditation you are simply coming back to your personal source of peace and relaxation. The low humming sound harmonizes the heart centre (fourth chakra) and brings you into contact with the love and peace that emanates from it. When you are centred in the heart, you automatically contact your inner peace. The heart transmits harmonic vibrations, which you experience as love and peace. Do this when you feel ill-at-ease with yourself, in the morning or evening, for 15–20 minutes.

Instructions

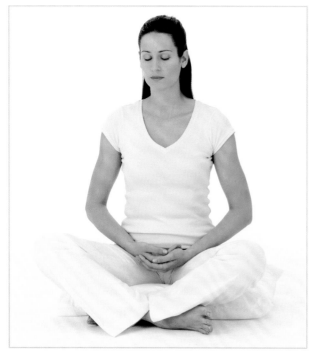

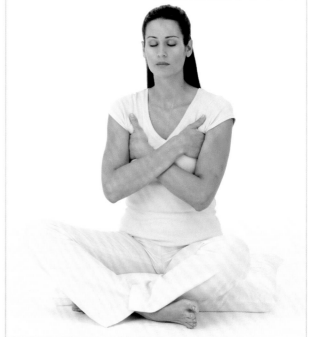

1 Sit (or lie) with eyes closed and your hands resting in your lap, or on your thighs. Breathe naturally in and out and make a deep humming sound on each out-breath. Maintain the same note. Do this for about 5 minutes, or longer if you wish.

2 Stop humming and place your left hand under your right armpit and your right hand under your left armpit, both thumbs exposed. Focus your attention on the chest area and let your heart become calm, with a feeling of love and peace rising from it. Do this for about 10 minutes. Alternatively, place both hands on the middle of the chest.

Mantra 'ohm' meditation

Mantras are Sanskrit syllables (words or phrases) that raise your state of consciousness. They are ancient and their origin is often unknown. Mantras are traditionally included in the daily practice of Buddhist prayer rituals. Sounds and mantras are used in meditation in order to activate the energy in the upper energy centres (chakras), to reach a higher vibration and consequently a higher level of consciousness.

The mantra 'ohm' (spoken as 'a-u-m') contains the ur-sound of the universe, and it is said that this sound is contained in everything. When chanting the mantra 'ohm' out loud, it feels as though the sound is entering your body and becoming one with it and everything else around you.

The meditation as a whole described below takes about 40–60 minutes.

Instructions

1 Sit comfortably, with your spine straight and your hands resting in your lap or on your thighs. Intone the 'ohm' mantra aloud, so that you start each syllable with your mouth wide open – 'a-u-m' – and end it in a hum, with your mouth closed. Do this on each out-breath, making it last as long as is comfortable.

2 Let the 'ohm' sound vibrate through your whole body. You can concentrate on the second chakra (belly area) and feel the vibration of the 'ohm' there. This will centre you. After a while you will feel that every cell in your body is filled with it. The more you feel deep harmony between yourself and the sound, the more you will feel yourself filled with a subtle sweetness. Do this for 20–30 minutes.

3 Now stop chanting 'ohm' and just sit silently for another 20–30 minutes. Feel the inner space and vibration this has created inside. You will feel energized, cleansed, rejuvenated and more aware.

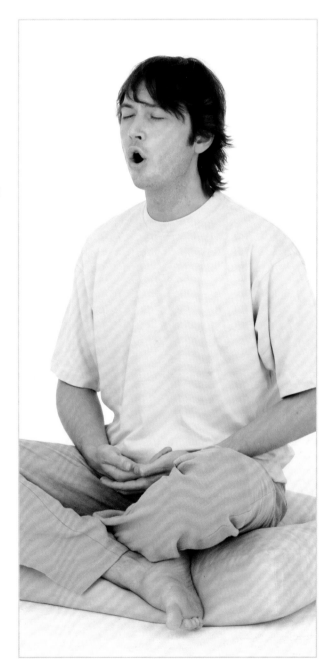

Hara centring

The 'hara' (or second chakra) is the best-known energy centre in the Eastern tradition, and the word comes from the Japanese. The hara point is located just below the navel. It is an important energy centre, as this is the point from which we receive life energy from the cosmos. You can do this meditation at any time of the day, particularly when you feel slightly off-centre or nervous about making a decision. The effect of this meditation is calm, self-trust and general centredness. The whole meditation takes about 20–30 minutes.

Instructions

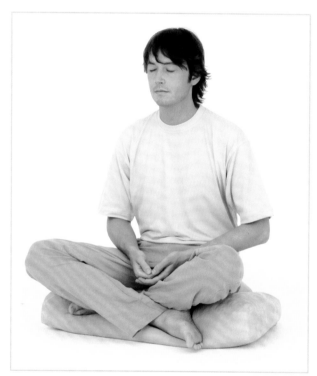

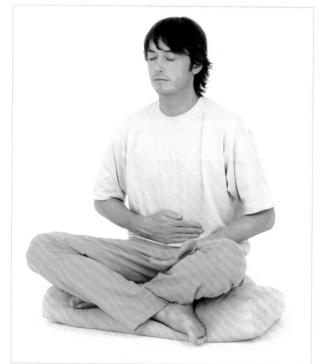

1 Sit comfortably, either on a chair or on the floor, with your spine straight. Keep your feet firmly on the floor and, if possible, your back unsupported. Place your hands, palms resting upwards, on your thighs. Keep your eyes closed. If you like, play soothing music to assist relaxation.

2 Connect with the hara (second chakra) point below the navel and visualize a line from here to the sixth chakra, between the eyebrows. Keep one hand on the hara to help you to hold your attention here.

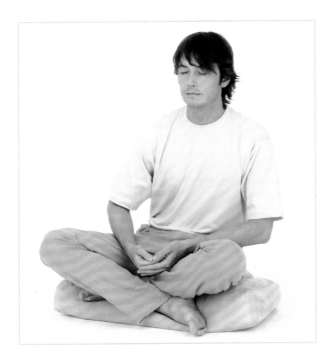

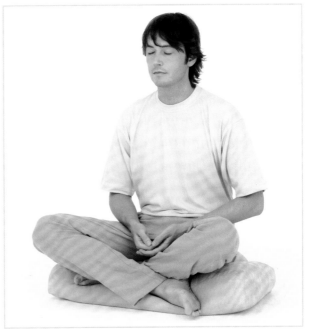

3 Now start moving your upper body anticlockwise in a circle for 10–15 minutes. While moving, keep your torso in a straight line from the hara (second chakra) point to the sixth chakra.

4 Let the circular movement become gradually smaller, until it stops completely. Be still and rest for about 5 minutes in an upright position, focusing on the energy in the hara.

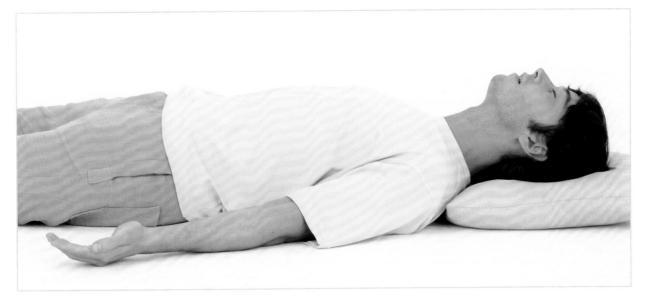

5 To finish the meditation, lie down on your back with your arms relaxed, palms facing upwards, legs slightly open and your mouth slightly ajar, jaw relaxed. Remain in this position for 5–10 minutes.

Atisha's heart-of-joy meditation

As soon as your body, mind and heart are functioning in harmony together, the heart opens and overflows with its own quality of joy. Joy contains pleasure and happiness for no apparent reason. It is like an overflow of life energy – whenever 'the cup is full', you are filled with something greater than you (ego). The key to finding such joy is connected on a deep level with your heart, as the heart naturally knows how to relax, enjoy and celebrate life.

This meditation comes from Atisha, an ancient Tibetan mystic. It is based on the understanding that the deeper we melt into the heart (or the heart chakra), the more we can disappear as a separate 'I'.

This technique teaches us to absorb anything that has been causing us suffering into the empty space of the heart. All these 'ghosts' – such as fear, worries, anxiety, struggles, feelings of unworthiness and judgements – are welcomed. As they enter the heart chakra when we breathe in, they dissolve and disappear into the empty space inside the heart. And once the heart has absorbed and transformed these negative energies, we can breathe out positive energies, such as love, joy and peace, sending them back into the body-mind-heart mechanism. The combination of Reiki with this meditation deepens the healing experience. Do this exercise for about 15 minutes, or as long as you like.

'I enjoyed all the meditations very much, in particular the one for the heart. I felt so much in touch with my feelings, with me really. Learning Atisha's heart meditation gives me the confidence and enables me to go deeper into myself. I feel I can trust now.'

Michaela

Instructions

1 Sit relaxed with your eyes closed. Take a few deep breaths and sigh on each out-breath. Place your hands on the middle of the chest area (the heart chakra) and connect with the heart.

2 Now bring to mind a current, or past, situation that has caused, or is causing, you suffering or pain. Breathe in and welcome the feeling. If tears come, just let them. Accept any emotion that arises and let yourself move deeply into the simple energy of the feeling, without any judgement of the mind.

3 Embrace the feeling and just be with it for a while, acknowledging it. Now ask the feeling, 'What do you need from me right now?' Wait for the answer to come.

4 After a period of time (perhaps 5–10 minutes), as you breathe out, reconnect with a feeling of peace, love or joy coming from your heart. Allow the out-breath to carry these blessings.

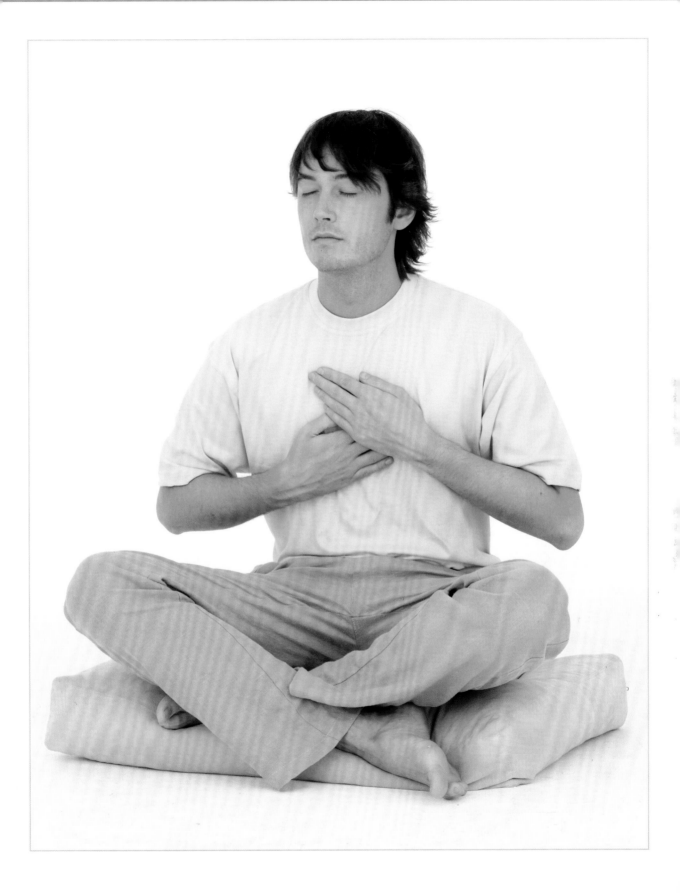

Relationship healing

We are all in a relationship with others: family, friends, colleagues and acquaintances. We may develop a special closeness and intimacy with a partner. But despite our longing to maintain a loving relationship, this is not always easy, as our needs and expectations differ from time to time. The willingness to understand the other person, and accept them the way they are, is one of the keys to regaining harmony in relationships. We all need to feel loved, and for intimacy to exist we need to be open to our partner, willing to share our thoughts, feelings and energy. The opening of our heart allows a natural flow of giving and receiving to take place.

Developing closeness

Do this exercise with someone you are close to, such as your partner. Try it when you feel you have missed quality time together recently or are feeling disconnected from one another. If you have had an argument and are ready to make up, this exercise helps you to become intimate again and to deepen your bond. Alternatively, try it prior to love-making, with the intention of experiencing your sexuality on a deeper level, suffused with feelings of love, tenderness, trust, caring and unity. Do this exercise sitting or lying down, facing one another, but do not talk during it. It takes about 15–20 minutes. Playing gentle music can help the relaxation, but is not vital.

Instructions

1 Sit comfortably face to face, close enough that you can easily reach your partner's chest. Use cushions to support your legs and back.

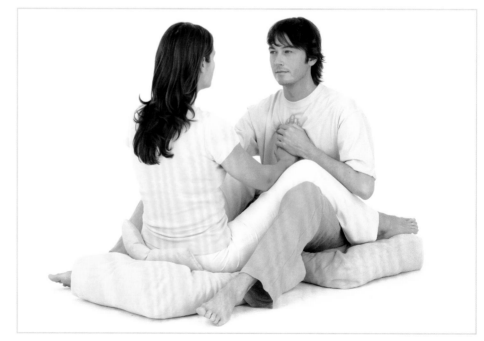

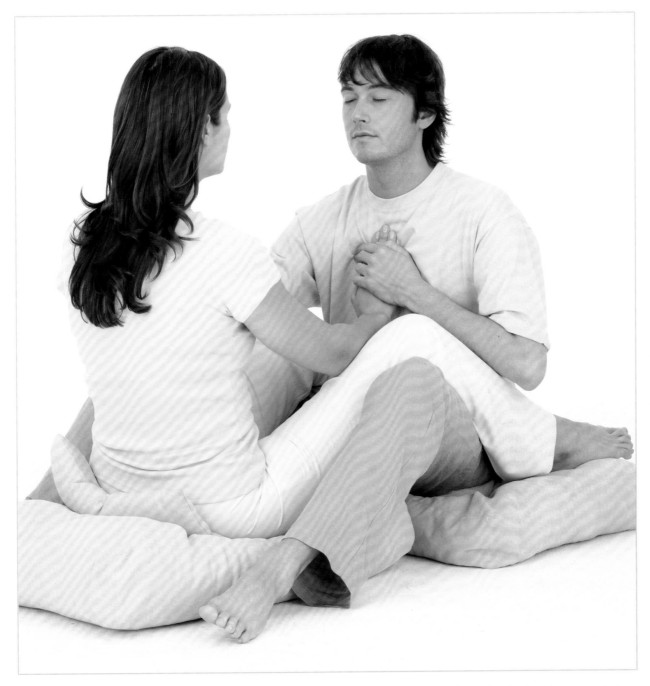

2 Both of you should place your right hand on your partner's heart centre (middle of the chest) and your left hand over their hand on your own chest. Keep your breathing relaxed and drop your chin. Allow the Reiki energy to flow into the chest area while gazing gently into each other's eyes.

3 While looking into each other's eyes, let 'the other' see you; and see 'the Buddha' (God or Christ) in the other. Continue in this way for about 2–4 minutes. If feelings such as tears or laughter arise, let them happen, and stay with the heart-connection.

4 Now both close your eyes. Be open to receive and feel the love and unity between you. Remain for as long as you like in this position, perhaps 10–15 minutes or longer. Alternatively, you can switch between eyes open and eyes closed; whatever feels right.

Talking and listening to your heart

The heart is our primary source of wisdom and understanding. It connects you to your intuition and knows your needs. You can talk to your heart as you would to an old and trusted friend and ask it about anything that burdens you, or anything for which you need a solution. Giving Reiki to the heart opens it up, and talking to it at the same time can be a deeply healing experience. This exercise helps you reconnect with your innermost feelings, and is a good way of releasing the worries and tensions of the day before going to bed. It will take about 15 minutes.

Instructions

1 Sit or lie down and take a few deep breaths. If you sense any tension in your body or heaviness in your heart, try sighing to gain some relief.

2 Place both hands on the heart centre (middle of the chest) and feel your heartbeat for a moment, focusing your attention on the fourth chakra, giving Reiki here.

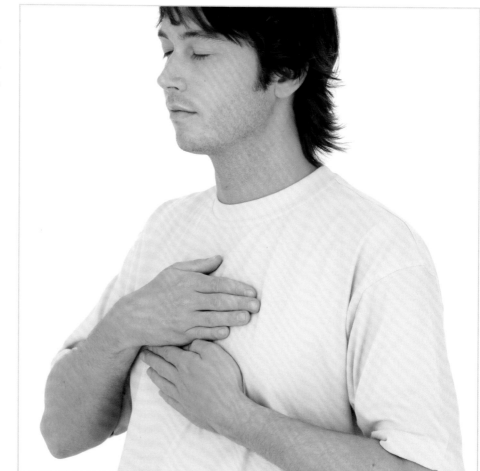

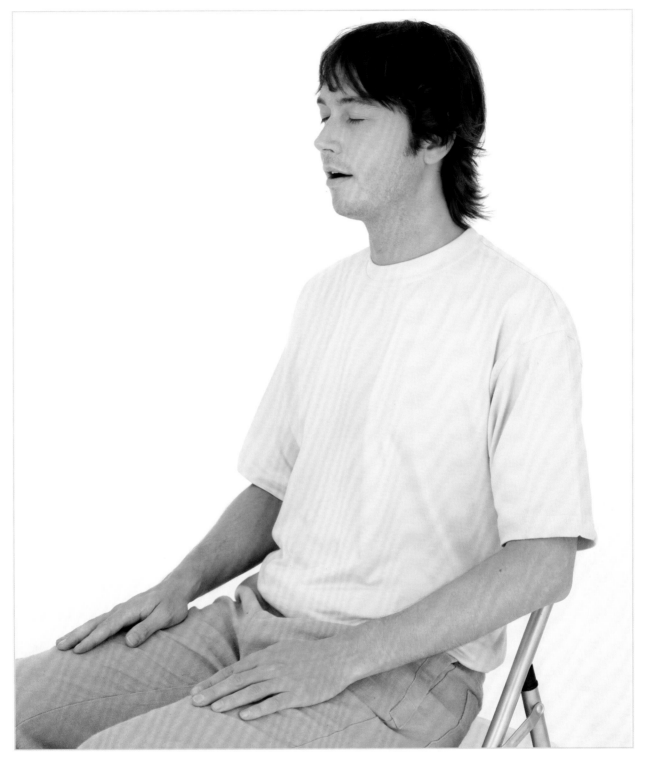

3 Now start talking to your heart as if it were an old friend. Ask it questions, such as: 'How are you?', 'Can I do anything for you?', 'What do you need from me right now?' or any question to which you need an answer.

4 Let any feeling that might arise just be there, and wait to receive answers from within.

Mood swings

When someone is in a bad mood, it is often difficult for them to change the feeling, although we all know that somehow 'this too will pass'. Treating a receiver's head with Reiki helps to increase the production of endorphins, the 'happiness hormones' of the body, and giving Reiki to the third chakra (the solar-plexus area) and middle back will reinforce their confidence and self-esteem. Allow a total of 15–20 minutes for this treatment.

Instructions

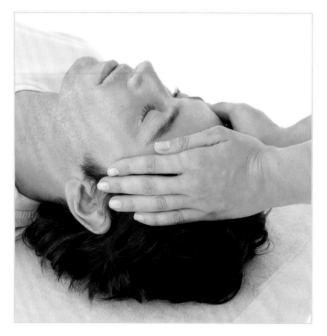

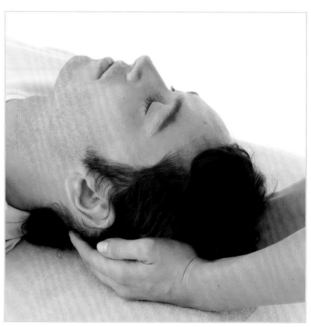

1 Place your hands on either side of the receiver's head, fingertips touching their temples, in Head Position Two. This position calms the mind and emotions.

2 Cup the back of the head with your palms, fingertips over the medulla oblongata, in Head Position Four. This position calms powerful emotions, strengthens intuition and brings clarity.

3 Place one hand on each side of the receiver's lower front ribcage. This treats the solar-plexus area, where many nerves end. It reduces fears and promotes relaxation.

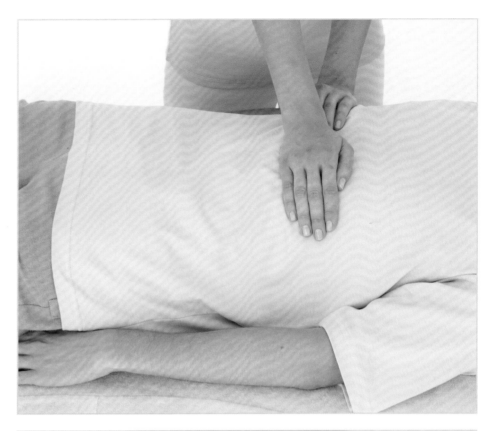

4 Now place your hands on the receiver's back above the waist at kidney height, in Back Position Three, to treat the kidneys, adrenal glands and nerves. This will help them let go of stress, fear and pain.

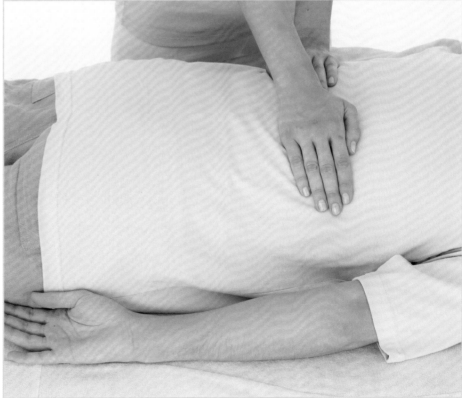

Boosting concentration

This exercise is especially useful before an exam, because it helps the receiver concentrate better and activates both the long- and short-term memory. It also helps ease stress and excessive mental activity. Hold each position for about 5 minutes, or longer.

Instructions

1 Once the receiver is either sitting or lying, place your hands over their eyes, forehead and cheeks, in Head Position One. This position helps energy to move back inwards and relaxes the eyes, which in turn affects the whole body.

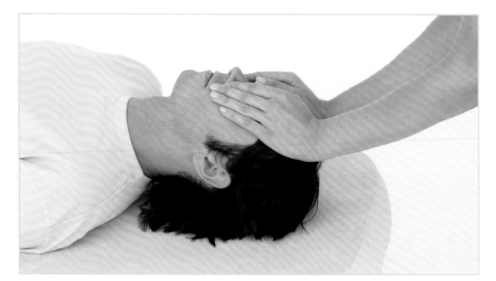

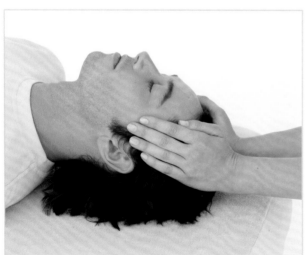

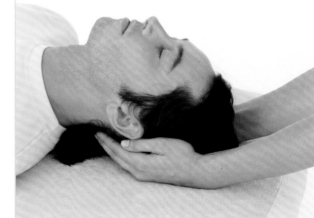

2 Now place your hands on either side of the receiver's head, your fingertips touching their temples, in Head Position Two.

3 Cup the back of the head with your palms, fingertips over the medulla oblongata, in Head Position Four. These last two positions balance the right (intuitive) and left (logical) sides of the brain, and help memory.

Emotional healing and balancing

This is a very nourishing treatment when someone is feeling low in energy or depressed, emotionally upset, worried or fearful. The hand positions balance powerful emotions, such as fear, confusion, shock and worry. Hold each position for 3–5 minutes. The whole treatment takes 40–60 minutes.

Instructions

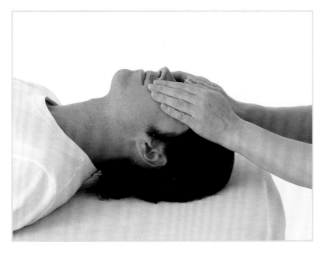

1 Lay your hands to the right and left of the receiver's nose so that they cover the forehead, eyes and cheeks, in Head Position One.

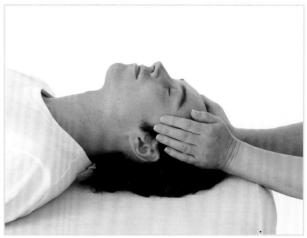

2 Lay your hands on both sides of the head, above the ears, with the fingertips touching the temples, and the palms following the shape of the head, in Head Position Two.

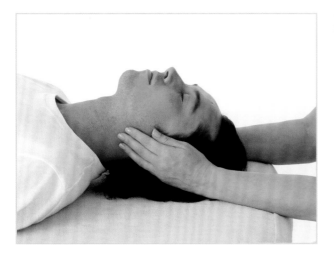

3 Lay your hands either side of the receiver's head over the ears, in Head Position Three.

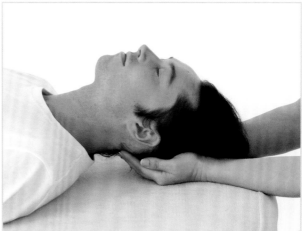

4 Cup the back of the head with the fingertips over the medulla oblongata, in Head Position Four.

5 Place one hand horizontally across the thymus gland, below the collarbone, and the other at right angles to the first, in the middle of the chest, in Front Position One. This position strengthens the heart and increases the capacity for love and enjoyment of life.

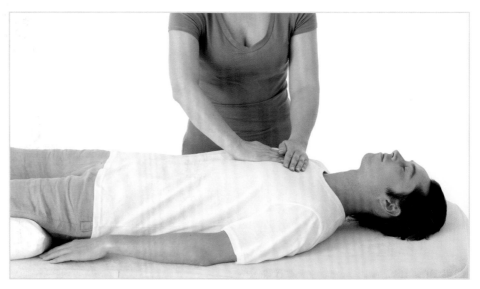

6 Place one hand on the lower abdomen just below the navel, and the other on the forehead. This position relaxes deep fears and helps the receiver let go of thinking, bringing the energy back to the centre of the body, the hara. Make a slow, circular hand movement around the navel, once or twice, to deepen the relaxation.

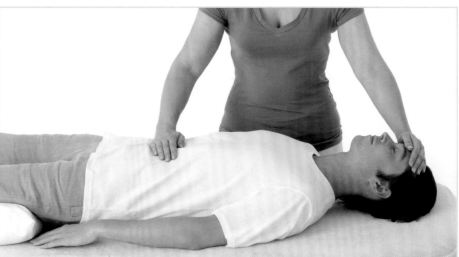

7 Now lay your hands flat on the inside of the receiver's thighs, between the upper legs, with your fingertips pointing in opposite directions. This helps to release deep-seated fears and emotions in the stomach area.

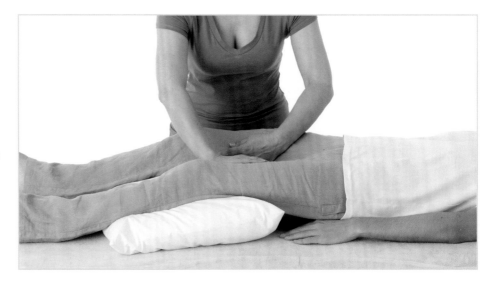

8 Place each of your hands on one of the receiver's knees. Giving Reiki here can release tension and fear, which may be held in the knees.

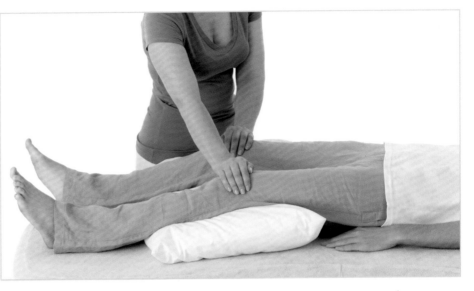

9 Now treat the back and place your hands on the lower ribs at kidney height, in Back Position Three. Treating this area helps the receiver to let go of the past and release stress and pain.

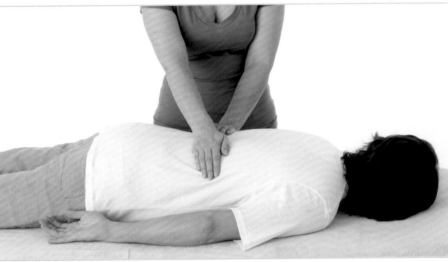

10 Place one hand on the receiver's lower back and the other on the medulla oblongata (between the head and the neck). This position gives a feeling of security and support.

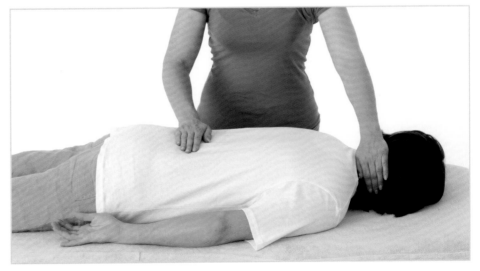

11 Lay your hands on the soles of the feet, ideally with the fingertips covering the toes, in Sole Position (A). Alternatively, rest the soft part of your palms on the toes and point your fingertips towards the heel, in Sole Position (B). This is good for strengthening the first chakra and grounds all the other chakras, too.

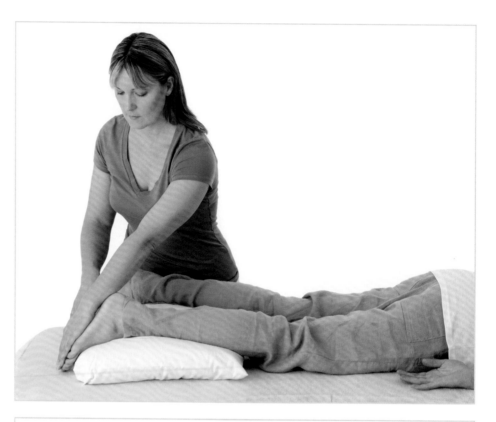

12 At the end of your treatment, smooth the receiver's aura from head to toe twice. Then draw an energy line (fingertips pointing towards the spine) from the base of the spine, up the spine and over the head. This strengthens the whole system. Allow the receiver to rest for a few moments.

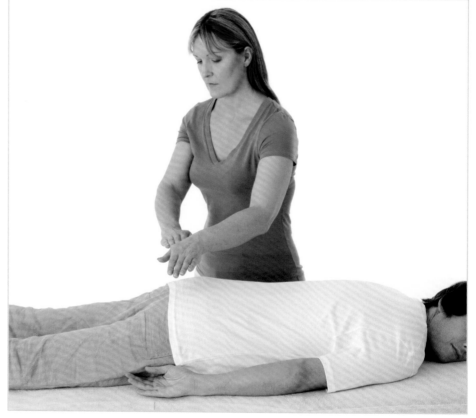

Emotional upsets

This is a short exercise for treating emotional upsets, especially during the menopause, as these hand positions also affect the release of hormones in the body. The pineal and pituitary glands are connected to the hypothalamus, which controls the release of hormones by nerve impulse. The following hand positions balance them, thus helping with emotional disturbances and problems with the body's temperature (good for menopausal hot flushes). This treatment takes 10–15 minutes.

Instructions

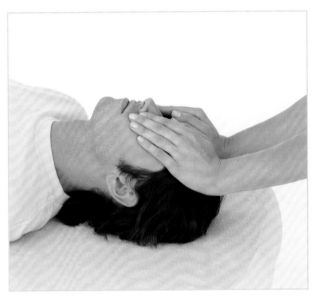

1 Cover the receiver's forehead, eyes and cheeks to relax their body, using Head Position One.

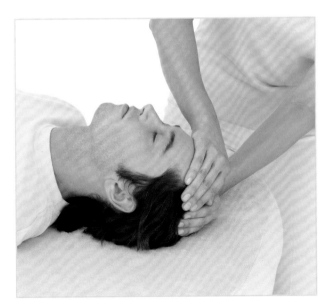

2 Lay your hands on top of their head horizontally, so that the outer edge of your lower hand touches the curve of the back of their head.

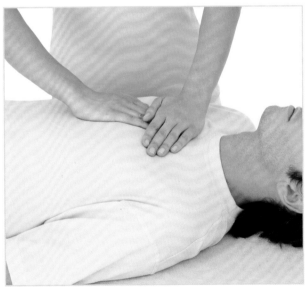

3 Additionally, lay one hand across the receiver's thymus gland, below the collarbone, with the other at right angles to the first on the breastbone, in the middle of the chest (together the hands should form a T). This Front Position One will reconnect them with a feeling of enjoyment of life.

Dealing with anger, frustration and depression

One of the most difficult feelings for many people to deal with is anger. Anger is a defensive reaction, often to the expectations or demands of others. The usual response is to become frustrated and to blame others. If anger does not have an outlet or acknowledgement, we tend to repress it and hold it in the body as an emotion of sadness or depression.

Depression is anger held back and turned, in a distorted way, onto the self. Reiki can help people first to recognize the underlying emotions, and then to balance and transform these negative feelings into positive ones. If

tears come, they should be allowed to flow. Keep your hands on the receiver in the position where the feeling started, until it dissolves; otherwise, keep them in each position for about 3–5 minutes.

Instructions

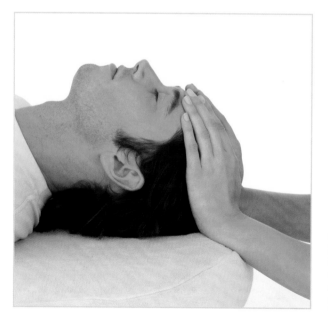

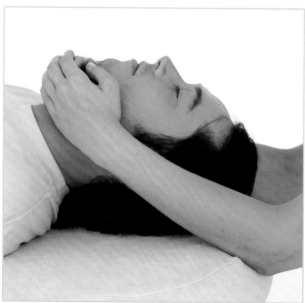

1 Lay both your hands on the top of the receiver's head, leaving a little gap between them to avoid the sensitive seventh-chakra area. This position helps centring and releases stress.

2 Now place your hands around the throat, in Head Position Five, without directly touching it. This is good for repressed anger and frustration, and promotes balanced self-expression.

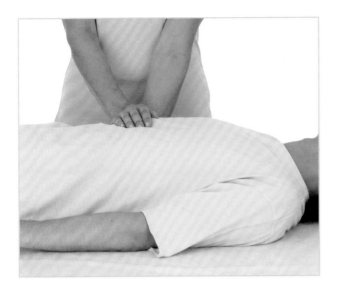

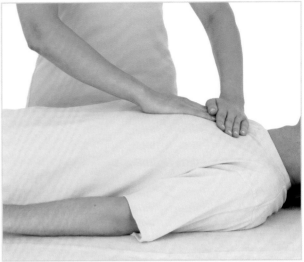

3 Place one hand on the left side of the receiver's lower front ribcage and the other opposite on the back, beneath the ribcage on the left side (in the 'sandwich' position), where the adrenals and kidneys are located. This calms the nervous system and strong emotions, and releases stress as well as pain. Now treat in the same way from the right side of the body: one hand on the lower right side of the front ribcage and the other under the middle back on the right side. This balances emotions such as anger and depression, and helps to reduce fear and frustration.

4 Lay one hand across the receiver's thymus gland, below the collarbone, and the other at right angles to the first on the breastbone, in the middle of the chest (the hands should form a T), in Front Position One. This position enables the emotional energies to come back into balance and increases the receiver's capacity for love and enjoyment of life.

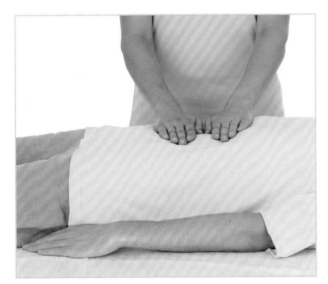

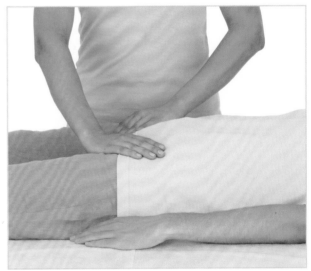

5 Lay one hand above and the other below the navel, in Front Position Four. This position has a strong calming effect and releases powerful emotions, such as fear, depression and shock.

6 Place both hands over the lower abdomen in the shape of a V, with your hands touching over the receiver's pubic bone (when treating a woman) or wider, with your hands over the groin area (when treating a man), in Front Position Five. This provides good grounding and helps fear of survival.

Life challenges

Everything is continually changing in life and we go through many different life stages between birth and death. Nothing is certain in life, except change, and the fact that material objects have no lasting substance. When we are going through difficult life phases, such as the menopause, a mid-life crisis or separation, we need to be open and to accept the challenge of change. All losses and changes offer us valuable opportunities to train ourselves to let go of old habits, patterns and thought processes.

When there is an unexpected event in our life, such as losing a life partner, we tend to react negatively. These negative emotions are like toxins in the body, and can cause 'dis-ease'. We need to become aware of negative emotions and transform them into positive qualities, such as understanding, patience, tolerance and forgiveness. Reiki can help this process by healing the areas that require most attention, on physical, emotional, mental and spiritual levels, thus transforming our responses to change and suffering. The pains of life and love are all stepping stones for our own growth towards liberation from suffering.

Easing separation

The end of a relationship usually brings immense change and uncertainty. We can feel disturbed by feelings of abandonment, bitterness, anger, guilt, fear of the future, sorrow and pain. However, these deep experiences of suffering and loss can also encourage us to take the first step on the path towards spiritual growth.

Reiki cannot necessarily help us to avoid a separation, but it can offer support during the process, helping us to separate in a loving way. It is important, and healing, to let go of any blame and anger we might still hold, and to forgive the other person for what they have done, asking them for forgiveness when we have wronged them. Reiki can help us transform negative feelings into a willingness to see our partner's beauty, love and uniqueness.

If separation is unavoidable, it is valuable to be kind and loving towards yourself. Reiki provides support for you in your sorrow and pain. If you can find time, give yourself a full Reiki treatment every day, for a while. Otherwise, try the following short treatment instead.

Maintain each hand position for about 3–5 minutes. The same hand positions can also be used to treat someone else, as described here.

Instructions

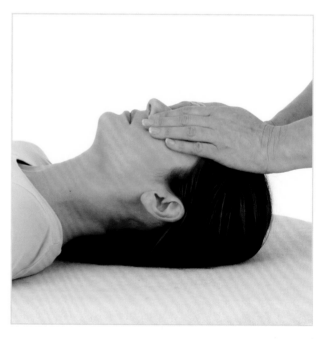

1 Lay your hands to the right and left of the receiver's nose, covering the forehead, eyes and cheeks, in Head Position One. This gives clarity of thought and intuition.

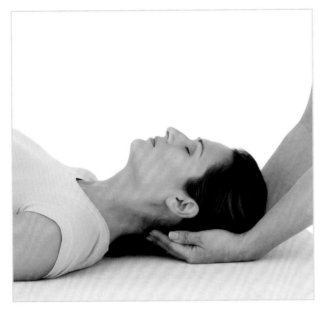

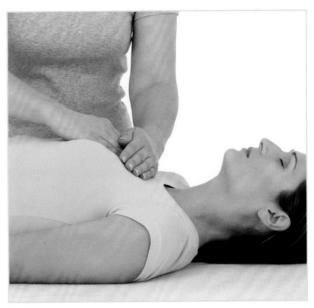

2 Cup the back of the head with the fingertips over the medulla oblongata, at the join between head and neck, in Head Position Four. This releases fear and any other strong emotions.

3 Lay one hand across the receiver's thymus gland, below the collarbone, and the other at right angles to the first on the breastbone, in the middle of the chest (with the hands forming a T), in Front Position One. This position supports enjoyment of life and the capacity to forgive.

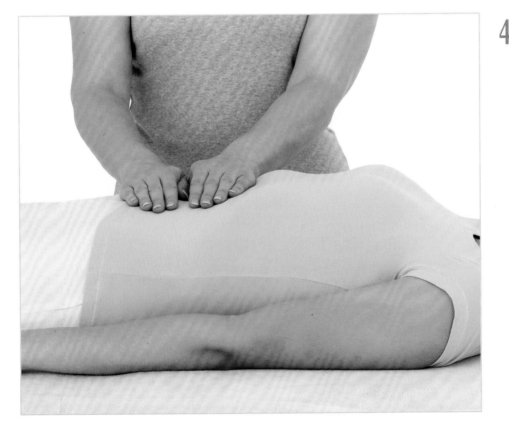

4 Lay one hand above the navel and the other below, treating the second and third chakras. This helps to ease fear, balance strong emotions as well as boost confidence.

Helping a mid-life crisis

The middle years are a turning point in life and represent a stage where we all have to face challenges of varying degrees. It can start any time between the ages of 40 and 50, when we become aware that half of our time on earth may have passed. Therefore, we start looking back on our life, reassessing the way we have been living. This gives us the opportunity to change our perspective. We may want to become more true to ourselves, and decide to use our remaining time and energy in life for what really interests, inspires and nourishes us – the things we always wanted to do. Reiki can help by providing us with the right energy, strength and trust to make significant changes. When you need inner guidance to make the right decisions, use the Self Mental Healing technique (see page 92).

Whenever you feel unsettled, immediately treat yourself with Reiki to improve your mood, self-confidence and outlook. Maintain each hand position for 3–5 minutes. The same hand positions can also be used to treat someone else.

Instructions

1 Place your hands over the pubic-bone area, in Front Position Four, to give energy to the first chakra, and to ground yourself and ease any fear of survival.

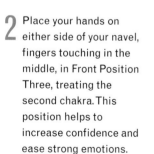

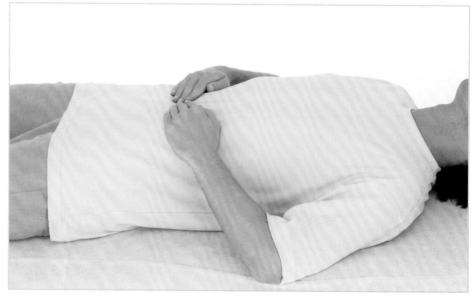

2 Place your hands on either side of your navel, fingers touching in the middle, in Front Position Three, treating the second chakra. This position helps to increase confidence and ease strong emotions.

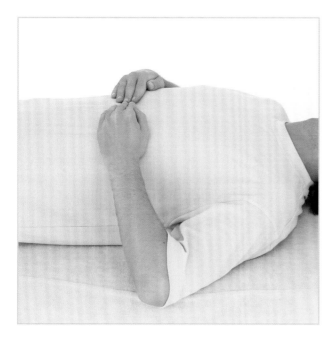

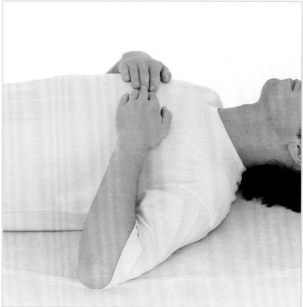

3 Place your hands on either side of your lower ribcage, fingers touching in the middle, in Front Position Two. This reduces fears and frustration, and promotes relaxation.

4 Lay both hands on either side of your chest, fingers touching just below the collarbone, in Front Position One, treating the fourth chakra. This increases the capacity for self-love and enjoyment of life.

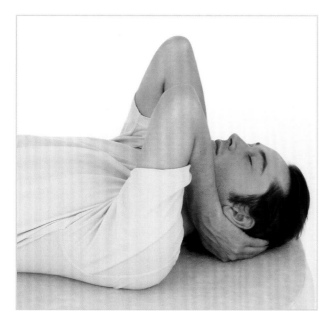

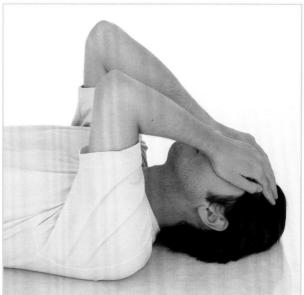

5 Lay your hands on the back of the your head, in Head Position Four, to calm the mind and any feelings of fear and anxiety.

6 Lay your hands over your eyes, covering the forehead, in Head Position One. This reduces stress, increases clarity and heightens intuition.

Helping relaxation

Many people find it difficult to relax fully. Relaxation cannot be forced; it happens by itself. In the personal healing process, the relaxation of body, mind and emotions plays an important role. As the body is near to the Self, conscious relaxation of the body is the first step. This makes it easier to achieve the second step, the calming of our thoughts, and, in the third stage, to allow positive feelings of love and peace, which provide deep relaxation and contentment. In moments of relaxation you are simply there, resting in your own energy. Your mind is still and your thoughts are not moving to future or past events. Your whole energy becomes very present, in the moment. Reiki is one method to help you become more relaxed. The flow of Reiki energy relaxes the body and mind, at the same time rejuvenating the whole body.

If you give yourself a daily full-body Reiki treatment, its rejuvenating effect will be noticeable. You are likely to look and feel more vibrant. It will also make you less susceptible to stress and will leave you with a deep sense of well-being. The full-body self-treatment takes 45–60 minutes (see page 128.) If you don't have that much available time, use this shorter version to treat yourself (or another person).

'Whenever I treat myself with Reiki, I feel a deep sense of inner peace and relaxation. Reiki is so very relaxing for the mind and the spirit, enabling me to go deeper into myself.'

Nigel

Instructions

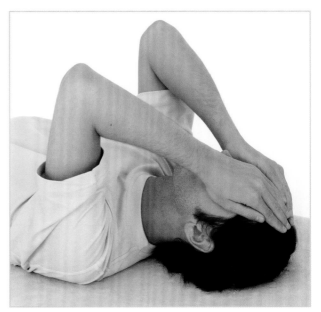

1 Place your hands over your eyes, resting your palms on the cheekbones, in Head Position One. Relaxing the eyes relaxes the whole body.

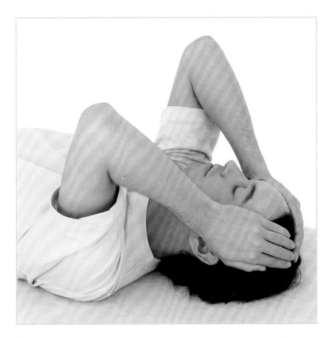

2 Place your hands on both sides of the head, above the ears, in Head Position Two. This harmonizes the left and right sides of the brain, having a calming effect on the conscious mind and easing depression.

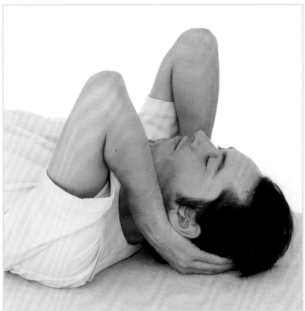

3 Cup the back of your head in both hands, fingers pointing upwards, in Head Position Four. This helps to calm powerful emotions, such as fear, worry, anxiety and shock.

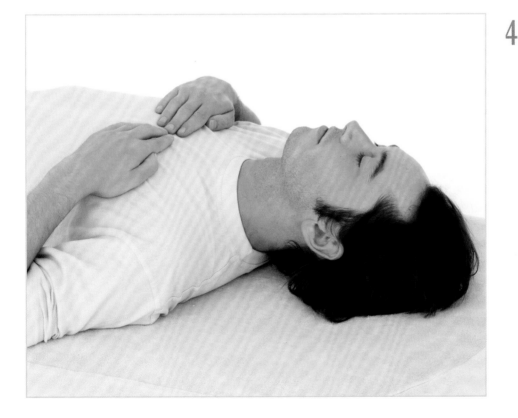

4 Lay your hands on either side of your upper chest, fingers touching just below the collarbone, in Front Position One. This encourages you to let go of negative feelings when you are weak or depressed. It also increases your capacity for love and enjoyment of life. (If treating someone else, use the T position on the front – see Step 5, page 224).

Stress prevention

Stressful situations are all too common in our fast-moving lives. The demands we place on ourselves and others, and the responsibility we feel, can cause stress symptoms such as headaches, migraines, shoulder and neck pain, upset stomachs, insomnia and anxiety attacks. In any stressful situation, the adrenal glands secrete hormones into the blood, which transports them all around the body, with harmful effects. Reiki balances your energies, strengthens your immune system and recharges your batteries quickly. It counteracts feelings of worry, restlessness or low spirits. You can do this treatment sitting on a chair, or lying down, as shown here. This treatment lasts for 15–20 minutes.

Instructions

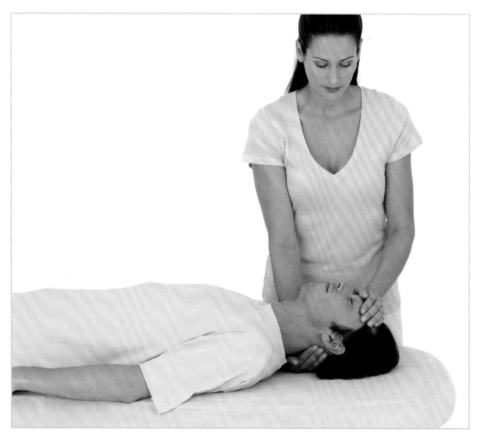

1 Place one hand on the receiver's forehead and the other on the back of the head over the medulla oblongata. This position helps to reduce stress and also facilitates meditation.

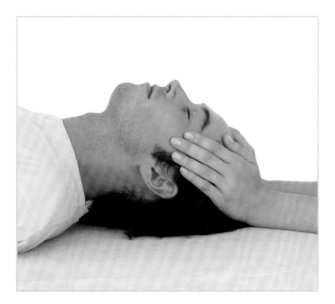

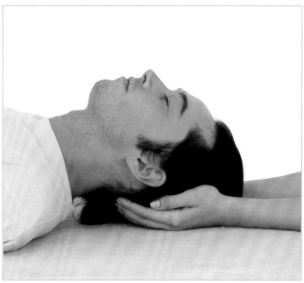

2 Lay your hands on either side of the head above the ears, in Head Position Two, with your fingertips touching the temples and palms following the curve of the head. This position treats the eye muscles and nerves, and balances the two sides of the brain.

3 Cup the back of the head in both hands, with your fingertips over the medulla oblongata, in Head Position Four. This treats the eye muscles and nerves, and balances both sides of the brain.

4 Additionally, treat the back and place your hands on the lower ribs at kidney height, in Back Position Three. Treating this area helps to let go of the past and release stress and pain.

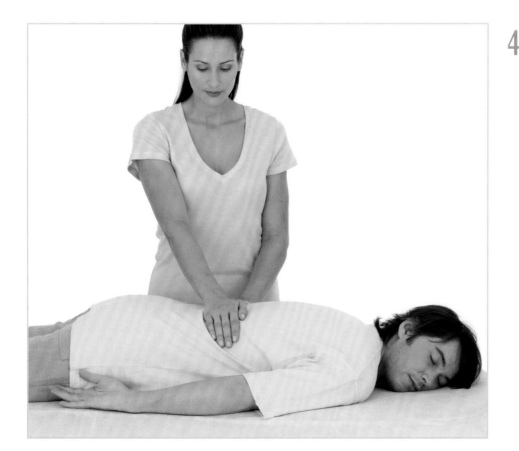

Boosting self-confidence

Use this treatment whenever you think it is important for you to feel secure and confident about yourself. You can do it simply to put you in a positive mood at the start of your day. The same hand positions can be used to treat someone else. Stay in each position for about 3–5 minutes.

Instructions

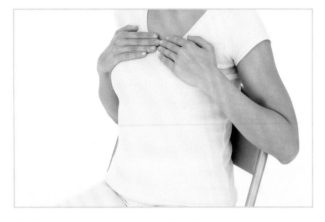

1 Place your hands on either side of your upper chest, fingers touching just below the collarbone, in Front Position One. This stimulates the heart centre, which can transform negative emotions into positive ones, such as love, trust and enjoyment of life.

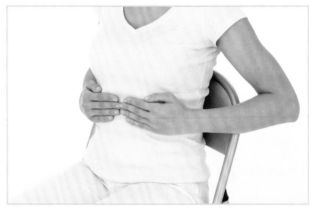

2 Place your hands over your lower ribcage, above the waist, fingers touching in the middle, in Front Position Two. This promotes relaxation and provides you with a feeling of trust when facing new situations.

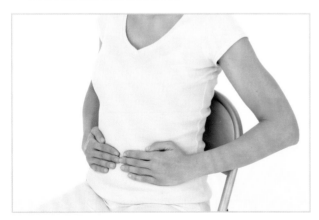

3 Place your hands on either side of your navel, fingers touching in the middle, in Front Position Three. This balances powerful emotions, such as fear, depression and frustration, as well as helping to increase self-confidence.

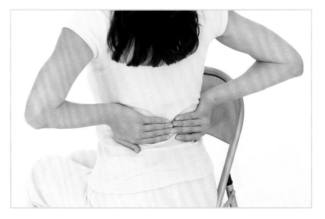

4 Place your hands around your waist at kidney height, fingers pointing towards the spine, in Back Position Three. This position alleviates stress and reinforces self-esteem and confidence.

Energetic and psychic protection

Reiki energy gives you protection from negative energies, but as you progress on your spiritual path with Reiki, you become more sensitive to other people's energies and more vulnerable and receptive to energetic and psychic draining. This is because, as the vibrational frequencies of your energy body are raised, they become more attractive to some of the lower energies. One possible outcome is that you are able to 'pick up' negative energies from other people and from your surroundings. It is a good idea to know how to protect yourself.

Creating a protective energy field

Both giver and receiver will be inside this auric energy field, and both will be surrounded by protective Reiki energy. If any negative energies are released by the receiver during treatment, they will not attach themselves to your energy field, but instead will be healed and transformed by the Reiki energy. This will only take about 5 minutes.

Instructions

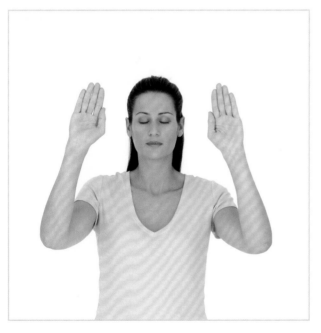

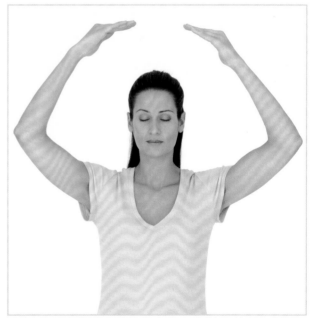

1 Start by 'drawing' the Power Symbol (see page 80) in front of you, then step into it and repeat its mantra (see page 79) three times. Use it with the intention that you will be protected from negative energies.

2 Now imagine yourself in a translucent bubble, or eggshell, of white or golden light. Visualize the Reiki flowing out of your hands, filling the space with healing white light. Additionally, imagine that the bubble or eggshell is closely surrounded by a fine mesh made of gold, which is penetrable only by love, light and Reiki.

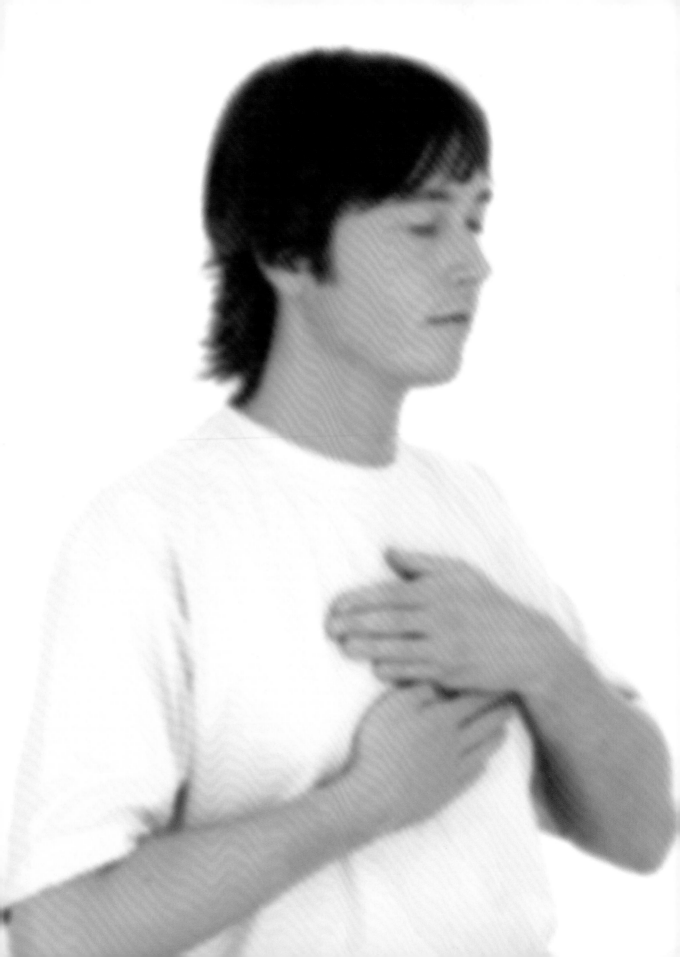

Becoming a Reiki practitioner

Now that you have developed your Reiki skills to a certain level – whether to the First, Second or Third Degree – you may well want to take this a step further and become a professional Reiki practitioner. The aim of this chapter is to help you focus on all the issues you need to consider and all the arrangements you need to make before you embark on this process.

Setting up a professional practice

If you are considering earning your living from giving Reiki treatment, you need to have progressed at least as far as the Second Degree and to have accumulated at least 70 hours of experience over a six-month period of time. It is also important to have experience of treating a wide range of ailments and issues, both physical and mental. You may have gathered this experience by starting off in modest ways (say, by treating close friends and family), but your aim now is to treat on a professional basis people whom you do not necessarily know. It is not essential to be a Reiki Master to set up as a professional Reiki practitioner.

Additional qualifications

Because Reiki healing works on the whole person, in mind, body and spirit, you need to learn how to ask the right questions (see also page 32) and to be a good listener. You may like to consider taking a counselling course to improve your listening skills. Co-counselling and Neuro-Linguistic Programming are two highly worthwhile disciplines that it would be worth investigating. You might also like to think about taking courses in energy work – such as work with chakras, psychic healing, meditation practice, heart opening and grounding work – as they will all contribute to your overall confidence as a practitioner and to your value as a Reiki healer. You will then be more effective in your work and your approach.

Informal groups

A good way to gather experience is to organize an informal Reiki group among your friends. You can do this either in your own home or in hired premises. You need a minimum of 4–6 people prepared to work on each other, either in pairs or as a group, and you can arrange a weekly (or fortnight or monthly) session in which you practise group Reiki exercises (see page 152) and paired healing sessions. You can create an enjoyable social session in which you may perhaps play relaxing background music, share food and drink (if appropriate) and exchange your thoughts and findings afterwards. Sharing Reiki with others makes you feel more connected and nourishes the heart.

Reiki and orthodox medicine

It is important to remember that Reiki is a complementary practice, so you should never use it as the sole healing method (see Cautions, page 246). If someone needs to see a doctor or receive medical treatment, and has not already done so, you must encourage them to make a visit to their doctor's surgery.

What sort of practice?

Depending on your availability and means, you need to decide what sort of practice you want to set up. Do you wish to start out by practising at home, or do you want to rent premises straight away? You may decide that working from home suits you better and fits in well with your other commitments. It may be a good way to begin in order to gain experience as a professional, and it may be the more economic option. If this is the case, then you need to have a suitable treatment room available in your home – ideally one that is not used for other purposes. It is important that this room is clean and quiet, and has a 'professional' atmosphere. Don't forget that if you use a room in your house for professional purposes, this will affect your household insurance.

Energetic cleansing of premises

You can use Reiki energetically to charge and cleanse rooms, particularly if you take over a new premises and they seem filled with negative energy. Amplify the Reiki energy by using the Power Symbol (see page 80) to cleanse the room's energy of negative influences and fill

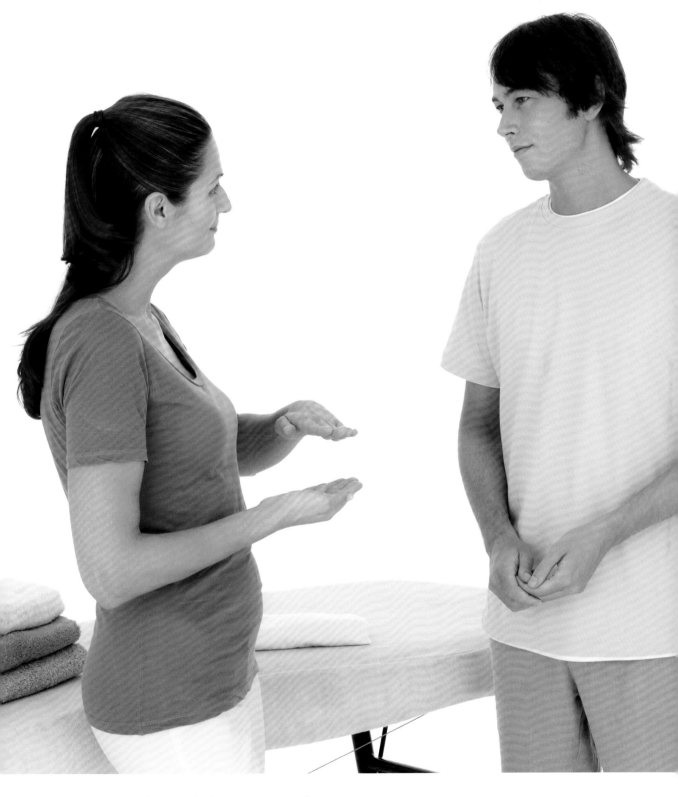

Before setting up a professional Reiki practice, you need to
ensure that you have the necessary skills and experience to
make a confident and effective healer.

it with harmonious vibrations. This is also a good way to cleanse the room before you start a treatment. In addition, you can use the Power Symbol on specific areas in the room where you want to enhance the flow of energy.

Assessing the market

Before embarking on becoming a professional, you need to think carefully about whether there is a need for your skills in your area. It is worth putting some effort into researching what other healers are already established in the vicinity, and whether the local population is receptive to what you have to offer. Visit doctors' surgeries, community centres, day centres, mother-and-toddler groups, playgroups, gyms, swimming pools, spas and leisure centres, hotels and guest houses, community facilities such as the town hall or library, local colleges and residential care homes as well as hospices and hospitals to see whether they allow healers to advertise on their notice boards.

Advertising your services

Think carefully about how you will contact potential clients and acquire a strong client base. Will you launch a professionally designed website, or will you print flyers to leave in local places such as the community centre, local college and natural health-food shops? Take care over the design of these things. Do they give the right impression? Bear in mind that your reputation will ultimately be made by word of mouth.

Charging appropriately

It is important to charge the same as other professional healers in your area. There is no point trying to undercut others with lower charges; your work will be undervalued by clients and other professionals will resent you.

Administration checklist

To set up professionally, you need to have a business head, to some extent. At the very least you must be organized and efficient, as well as being a good Reiki healer. It may be worth the expense to employ an administrative assistant who can keep an appointment book and records of clients, answer the phone while you are treating people and keep things neat and tidy.

You are running a small business, so you may need to engage the services of an accountant, who will require access to your business records and bookkeeping at the end of the financial year. You should keep running records of all the costs you incur, including: electricity, rent, equipment and stationery expenses, advertising and outreach costs, travel, client fees, employment costs and postage and telephone expenses, plus the cost of further courses and qualifications, if relevant. You also need to be insured for professional indemnity and public liability; contact the Reiki Association or the UK-Reiki Federation for further information (see page 251 for full contact details). All expenses incurred are tax-deductible, so you must keep all your receipts.

Equipment and ambience

Your treatment room need not be large, but it should contain the following items as standard: a professional massage table (folding/portable versions are available); two chairs (one for yourself and one for the client); a desk for your computer, notes and records; cushions and pillows; a shawl; a blanket; a box of tissues. Remember that confidentiality is the key to establishing a relationship of trust with the client, so all record-keeping should be kept securely. Keep all your professional qualification certificates on display in your treatment room or waiting area.

The room should be warm and cosy, perhaps with a colourful rug on the floor. If you like, you can use a few scented candles to create soft lighting, and some house plants to add greenery. Wall decorations, such as meditation mandalas, should be tasteful and discreet, and background music should be soothing and low-key. If you wish, keep a picture of Usui or a favourite spiritual teacher or guru in your treatment room. You might want to consult a Feng Shui expert to ensure that all the elements of your room are auspiciously positioned in relation to its shape and layout. If space permits, provide a waiting area for clients.

Whether you work from home or rent premises, choose a calming decor, with harmonious colours and simple decorations to create a friendly yet businesslike atmosphere. If working from home, you must make sure that neither you nor the client is disturbed by pets, children, ringing phones and so on; if you are charging for your services, clients will expect a high level of professionalism. If funds permit, you may be able to rent suitable premises, either by yourself or as part of a practice with other healers.

Demonstrations, workshops and health fairs

You may have the opportunity to give talks, facilitate workshops and conduct demonstrations. These are skills well worth acquiring, since they help you to reach a wider audience, promote you as a healer and build up your client base. Being 'on show' in this way may seem daunting initially, but a few simple presentation skills and

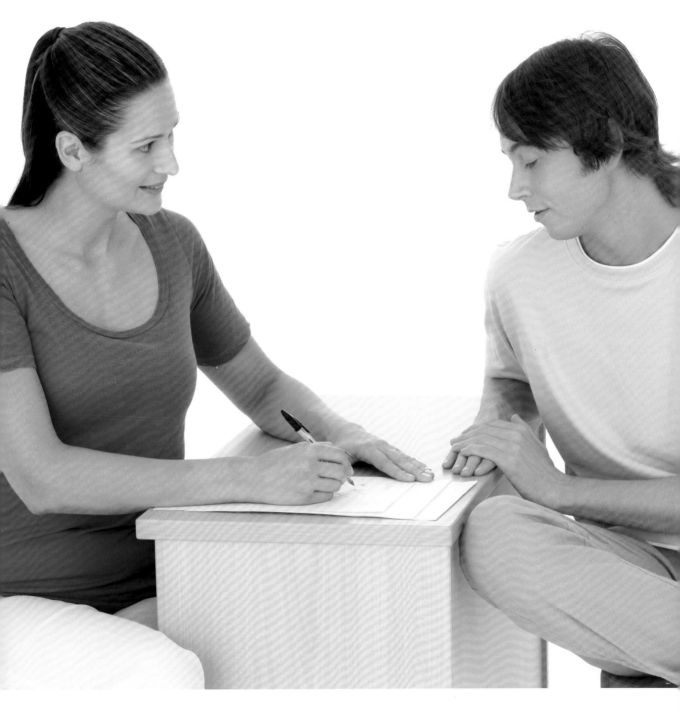

plenty of practice will quickly make an expert of you. Take the time to plan your presentation by making a crib sheet to consult occasionally while you are speaking, and then try to make eye contact with your audience, while speaking in as natural and relaxed a fashion as possible. Speak from your heart and you will sound knowledgeable, authentic and trustworthy.

Make sure that you establish the right ambience at your practice – it needs to be reassuringly welcoming, comfortable and calming yet efficient and businesslike.

Remember to outline the basics of how Reiki works: it is a natural hands-on healing skill that is enhanced and strengthened by the use of special symbols, and works in the energy body via the chakra system. Outline a selection of the ordinary ailments that Reiki can help to heal. Be aware that some of your explanation may sound outlandish to people who have not come across Reiki before, so be prepared to explain everything simply and in a common-sense way.

Afterwards, give a short demonstration with a volunteer to show people how Reiki works in practice, using a variety of the normal hand positions, or choose some positions from the short Reiki treatment (see page 147), given on a chair. Be as open as possible about what Reiki is, and answer any questions frankly and honestly. Counter any awkward questions in a friendly fashion. Use humour if the audience responds favourably to it. At the end, have a supply of flyers and/or business cards ready to hand out to those who are interested, and offer to answer individual questions.

Your client and you

The client/practitioner (healer) relationship is a special one. When you establish a client/practitioner relationship, you are held in a position of trust and you must act, at all times, with the highest standards of integrity. You should never touch a client inappropriately or unnecessarily. Remember that some of the Reiki hand positions concern intimate parts of the body, and advice is given earlier in the book on how to carry these out correctly for both men and women (see pages 133, 137, 150, 174 and 184). Remember that there is no need for your client to remove any clothing except shoes, belts and jewellery.

Be very clear about the boundaries between client and practitioner. Never take advantage of such a relationship and start a sexual relationship with a client. This implies a 'misuse of power' and will always reflect negatively on you, showing a lack of integrity and professionalism.

You may find that clients occasionally become upset during treatment, especially when emotions (sadness, anger, grief, etc.) are aroused. Stay centred and calm, and continue treating in the same hand position as when the emotions first showed. Encourage the client to express their feelings, and create a safe space for them to feel accepted and loved the way they are right now. Discretion and confidentiality are part of your role as a professional practitioner. Never talk to another person about anything regarding your client's personal issues and privacy.

To protect yourself from energy-draining during treatment, use the exercise on creating a protective energy field (see page 239). Reiki energy in itself gives you protection from negative energies, but as you refine your energy bodies, you also become more receptive to energetic and psychic drains. This means that you could absorb negative energy from your client. After the treatment, always wash your hands up to the elbows in cold water, because cold water also clears energies.

Length of sessions/courses of treatment

You should aim to treat each client for about an hour, adding another 15 minutes for a question-and-answer session at the beginning, and allowing for your note-taking and record-keeping and an advisory session after the treatment is completed (thereby totalling a maximum of one and a half hours). It is important that the client feels relaxed and unrushed by time constraints. You may recommend that he or she comes to you for a series of four initial treatments over a few weeks, but the client should not feel obliged to carry this many treatments out, as it may represent an expense that cannot easily be met. Ideally, after the first four initial sessions, the client should continue with Reiki until the energy is balanced, and healing and wholeness are restored, which might take 6–12 treatments.

CAUTIONS

- Do not try to diagnose what is medically wrong – leave that to a qualified medical practitioner.
- Whenever you notice during treatment that an organ or an area in the client's body is feeling weak, or taking unusual amounts of energy in, consider recommending to the client a visit to their doctor to have it checked out.
- Do not give any healing promises with Reiki.
- Do not recommend that the client only receives Reiki, or switches completely from seeing an orthodox doctor to just practising Reiki.
- Instead suggest other medical care or healing disciplines that you think may be helpful and appropriate for the client.
- Always ask the client whether they have checked with their doctor that it is all right for them to receive Reiki treatment.

Using Reiki with other disciplines

Reiki can be used in conjunction with a number of other healing therapies, and especially with those that involve hands-on techniques. It brings additional power to any form of healing-touch technique and flows automatically from healer to receiver. Reiki can be combined successfully with massage, shiatsu, acupuncture, acupressure, chiropractic, Aura Soma colour therapy, Bach Flower Therapy, homeopathy, breath therapy, polarity, Rolfing, cranio-sacral therapy, hypnosis, foot reflexology, aromatherapy, cosmetic massages and many other complementary healing techniques. Some Reiki practitioners also work in the fields of massage and aromatherapy, and report that their work has positively changed and intensified since taking the First Degree.

Massage

Reiki is ideal for combining with massage. However, Reiki is not itself a massage technique and you should not apply any pressure or use a circular motion when carrying it out.

If you are a professional masseuse, try the following techniques. At the start of the massage, begin with Head Position One (see page 134) to relax the receiver and direct energy inwards. Then massage the sides of the throat and nape of the neck for a few minutes. Also massage the medulla oblongata area and along the back of the head. Next, use Head Position Four (see page 135) and hold the head. After a few minutes, you may notice how the receiver relaxes deeply and lets go of tension. Now carry out a complete head and face massage as you usually do.

Then lay your hands in Head Positions Two and Three (see pages 134–135) and let Reiki energy flow. Now massage the whole front of the body, working from head to toe. Let your hands rest between massage strokes. Work your way to the feet. Then ask the receiver to turn over and work upwards along the backs of the feet and

Reiki combines well with other hands-on healing techniques, such as massage. Many therapists supplement and intensify their work with Reiki energy.

legs. After you have massaged the back, treat the back of the body with Reiki. Use Back Positions One to Five (see pages 138–139). Lastly, treat the knees and lay your hands on the soles of the feet.

Hypnosis

Hypnosis and Reiki complement each other well. A Reiki treatment can be given before, during or after a hypnosis session, which simplifies the awareness of events in the past, present and future. Conversely, a Reiki full-body treatment can be greatly intensified by hypnosis, as you relax more quickly and profoundly in the hypnotized state. If you have learnt a self-hypnosis technique, you will enjoy a new experience with Reiki. Make a recording of your own voice for the hypnosis lead-in and then treat yourself directly. You can also use the combined effects of hypnosis and Reiki to concentrate on certain topics. The combination of Reiki and hypnosis is particularly suitable for addressing depression, withdrawal symptoms from addictions, childhood traumas, eating disorders and various psychosomatic complaints.

Meditation

Using Reiki, you can enter a wonderful state of meditation. Reiki simply touches deeper layers within, and puts you in touch with the core of your being. Here you contact your source and feel connected with the whole. You can use the Power Symbol (see page 80) to bring greater awareness to your meditation. By doing this, you create a higher vibration of light energy in and around you, making it easier for you to raise the level of your consciousness and to observe your body, thoughts and feelings. In meditation you let go and relax. You let yourself fall into your innermost being – it is a state of absence of wanting and an absence of doing.

Bach Flower Therapy

This therapy was developed in the 1930s by English physician Dr Edward Bach, who explored the healing effect of the flowers of certain plants. He established that they can harmonize conflicts on the mental–spiritual plane. By a simple and natural method, he was able to capture the energy frequencies of flowers and conserve them in a flower essence. He then observed that illnesses caused by emotional imbalance or a false mental attitude disappeared shortly after the patient took these specific flower essences.

Reiki can help the process by enriching the essence with Universal Life Energy. Because Reiki energy (just like the flower essence) consists of subtle vibrations, these two methods support each other perfectly. You hold the Bach-remedy treatment flask in one hand and lay the other hand over it, with your fingers closed. Let Reiki energy flow into the flask for a few minutes. Use the Power Symbol (see page 80) to make the mixture even more effective.

Aura Soma colour therapy

This holistic therapy combines the healing effects of colours, plants, precious stones and perfumes, and was devised by English pharmacist Vicky Wall, who was blind. She received the inspiration for the first Aura Soma essences while in a meditative state. Unable to see the brilliant colours that appeared when she mixed the ingredients together, she discovered that they produced intense vibrations.

Reiki and Aura Soma make a good combination. You can choose an appropriate essence at the start of every Reiki treatment for smoothing the receiver's aura (see page 62). After the treatment, you can also cleanse yourself energetically using an essence. In Reiki seminars, especially before an energy-transmission, it is helpful to cleanse the aura with Aura Soma essences.

MEANINGS OF THE DIFFERENT COLOURS OF AURA SOMA ESSENCES

Choose the essence (Pomander or Quintessence) intuitively or according to what is appropriate to the needs of the receiver.

Green For finding inner space, cleansing and centring
White For bringing in light, renewal and cleansing
Red For grounding, revitalizing and protection
Yellow For bringing back sparkle (when fearful)
Orange For absorbing shock and bringing insights
Turquoise For creative communication of the heart
Blue For inner peace and inner sight
Pink For self-love, warmth and caring
Gold For reconnecting with innate wisdom
Violet For calming and healing
Deep magenta For compassion and deep caring
Deep red For grounding and deep protection

Reiki makes a powerful contribution to meditation, enabling you to connect with your innermost self. Using the Power Symbol will enhance your awareness still further.

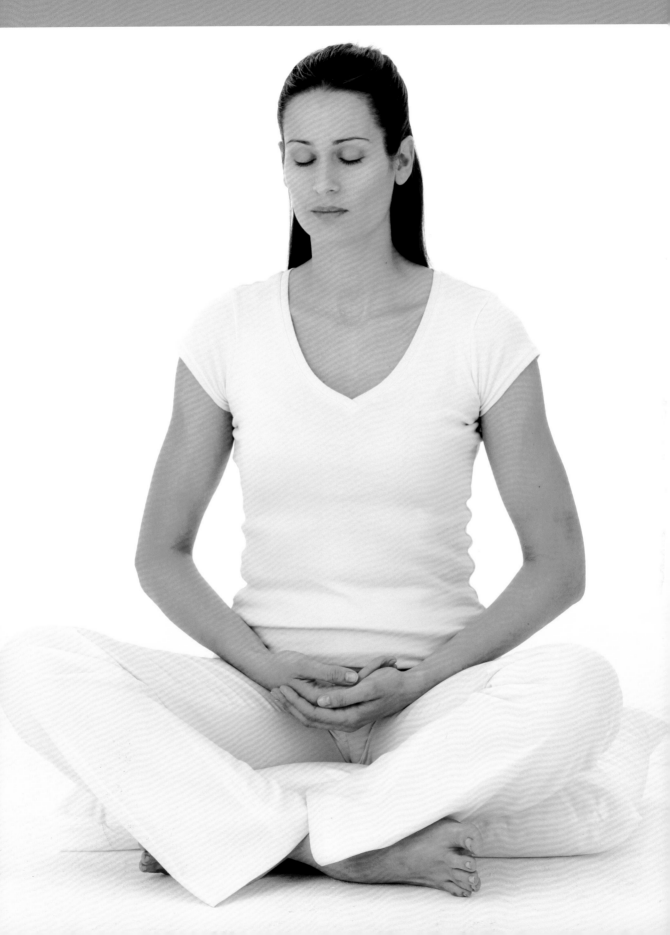

Afterword

The Reiki healing system uses energy-transmission to raise the vibratory rate of our physical and energy bodies. We are able to let a higher energy force flow through us. This not only affects us, but also our surroundings, and heightens the vibratory rate of the planet.

Reiki and the evolution of consciousness

We are living in a very important time on our planet earth. It is an awesome thought that we may not be able to survive if we continue to pursue our present hostility and profit-oriented, exploitative behaviour between countries, religions and people. We need to wake up to a new consciousness, which vibrates at a higher level of energy – the energy of love and healing. We can choose to work together, support each other and not exploit Mother Earth. It is time to shake off old beliefs and patterns of thinking, and the behaviour of isolation and hostility. We can decide to be more caring towards each other so that we feel we are one world.

Up to now, most of humanity has been caught up in dysfunction; a feeling of separation from our divine essence. Reiki power is an essential tool that can help us reconnect with our resources and return us to our true essence. Each healing, on a deeper level, means a 'return'; and the meaning of self-healing is to return to your true nature – your essence.

The Reiki method facilitates enhanced intuition and connection to our Higher Self, and we are able to gain a wider and purer view. We can glimpse that we are not separate – neither from our divine essence nor from another's divine essence; we are all one. This knowing brings immense comfort and blessings, and heals the whole world.

My wish is that this book has given you insights, inspiration and guidance for your own life, as well for healing our planet. We are all part of its aliveness, which expresses itself through humans, animals, plants and nature. We need to acknowledge that we belong to nature and to life itself, and are a part of this unfolding wonder.

Through Reiki we can wake up to a new consciousness and reconnect with our precious resources – those that are within us as well as those that surround us.

'How spiritual you are has nothing to do with what you believe, but everything to do with your state of consciousness. This, in turn, determines how you act in the world and interact with others.'

From A New Earth *by Eckhart Tolle, contemporary spiritual teacher*

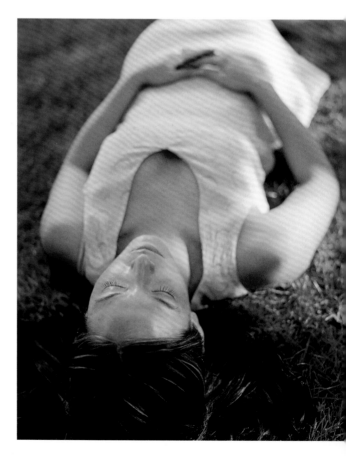

Appendices

Recommended reading

Inner Reiki – A practical guide for healing and meditation, Tanmaya Honervogt, Gaia Books (2001)

A New Earth – Awakening to your life's purpose, Eckhart Tolle, Dutton (2005)

Reiki for Emotional Healing, Tanmaya Honervogt, Gaia Books (2006)

Reiki: Healing and harmony through the hands, Tanmaya Honervogt, Gaia Books (1998)

Reiki To Go – Simple routines for home, work and travel, Tanmaya Honervogt and Carol Neiman, Gaia Books (2005)

Recommended music and guided CDs

Tanmaya has created a range of CDs for guided Reiki self-treatment and meditation:

Heal yourself with Reiki – 18 stages for self-healing

Inner Healing (with music by Deva & Miten) – 11 stages for self-healing

Reiki-Wellbeing (with music by Deuter) – 3 short Reiki self-treatments (rejuvenating energy; balancing chakras; helping with sleep)

Useful addresses and websites

International House of Reiki, PO Box 9, Glebe 2037, Sydney NSW, Australia

Morning Peninsula Reiki Centre, www.geocities.com/tradreikivic

The Reiki Alliance – Germany, www.reiki-alliance-deutschland.de/

The Reiki Alliance – USA, www.reikialliance.com/

The Reiki Association, www.reikiassociation.org.uk/

Reiki Outreach International, PO Box 191156, San Diego, CA 92159-1156, USA, www.annieo.com/reikioutreach

Reiki Outreach International, PO Box 326, D-83090 Bad Endorf, Germany, www.roi_d@topmail.de

The UK-Reiki Federation, PO Box 71, Andover, Hampshire SP11 9WQ, UK, www.reikifed.co.uk

Index

Acknowledgements

I want to thank Rajen – Peter Campbell (my life long friend) for always being there when I had queries about the text and giving me valuable feedback during the process of writing. Many thanks to Jo Godfrey-Wood (my editor of many years working together now), who understands so well the method, the spiritual side and depths of Reiki. I would also like to thank all my Reiki students in England (especially Krissie for modelling) and Germany for their trust and who have shared with me their Reiki healing experiences and allowed me to use them in this book.

Tanmaya can be contacted at:
P.O. Box 86
Crediton
EX17 6WU
Tel: 01363-83870
www.tanmaya.info

The UK Reiki Federation can be contacted at:
P.O. Box 71
Andover
Hants
SP11 9WQ
Tel: 0870-8502209
www.reikifed.co.uk

The publisher would like to thank Bonnie Fraser of Alternative Products Limited for supplying the Starlight massage table and the therapist's stool used in the photography. For more information visit: http://www.apl-starlight.com/.

Special Photography:
© Octopus Publishing Group Limited/Ruth Jenkinson
Models Michelle Liebetrau and Tony Craig at Modelplan and Kristina Streatfield.

Other Photography:
Alamy/JTB Photo Communications Inc. 13; /Pedro Del Rio 20.
Corbis/Bloomimage 158, 208; /Michael A. Keller 162; /Scott Wohrman 21.
Getty Images/Martin Barraud 29; /Tony Metaxas 22; /Walther Bear 23.
Octopus Publishing Group/Frazer Cunningham 65; /Mike Good 72, 73, 153, 154, 155; /Mike Prior 133; /Paul Bricknell 117; /Peter Pugh-Cook 50; /Russel Sadur 51, 67; /Russell Sadur 71, 115, 204, 205.
Photolibrary/Rebecca Emery 250.
Science Photo Library/Francoise Sauze 18.
Page 15 courtesy of **www.shiva-parvati-institut.de**

Executive Editor Jessica Cowie
Project Editor Charlotte Macey
Executive Art Editor Leigh Jones
Designer Peter Gerrish
Illustrator KJA Artists
Picture Research Manager Giulia Hetherington
Senior Production Controller Simone Nauerth